The Other Family Doctor

The Other Family Doctor

A Veterinarian Explores What Animals
Can Teach Us About Love, Life, and Mortality

Karen Fine, DVM

⚓

ANCHOR BOOKS

A DIVISION OF PENGUIN RANDOM HOUSE LLC

NEW YORK

AN ANCHOR BOOKS ORIGINAL 2023

Copyright © 2023 by Karen Fine

All rights reserved. Published in the United States
by Anchor Books, a division of Penguin Random House LLC,
New York, and distributed in Canada by Penguin Random
House Canada Limited, Toronto.

Anchor Books and colophon are registered
trademarks of Penguin Random House LLC.

The Library of Congress has cataloged the Anchor Books edition as follows:
Names: Fine, Karen R., author.
Title: The other family doctor : a veterinarian explores what animals can teach us
about love, life, and mortality / by Karen Fine.
Description: New York : Anchor Books, 2023.
Identifiers: LCCN 2022008682 (print) | LCCN 2022008683 (ebook)
Subjects: LCSH: Fine, Karen R. | Veterinary medicine—Massachusetts—
Anecdotes. | Veterinarians—Massachusetts—Anecdotes. | Veterinarians—
Massachusetts—Biography.
Classification: LCC SF613.F5288 A3 2023 (print) | LCC SF613.F5288 (ebook) |
DDC 636.089092 B—dc23
LC record available at https://lccn.loc.gov/2022008682
LC ebook record available at https://lccn.loc.gov/2022008683

Anchor Books Hardcover ISBN: 978-0-593-46689-6
eBook ISBN: 978-0-593-46690-2

Book design by Nicholas Alguire

anchorbooks.com

Printed in the United States of America
10   9   8   7   6   5   4   3   2   1

To my father, who taught me the meaning of family,
and my grandfather, the finest family doctor

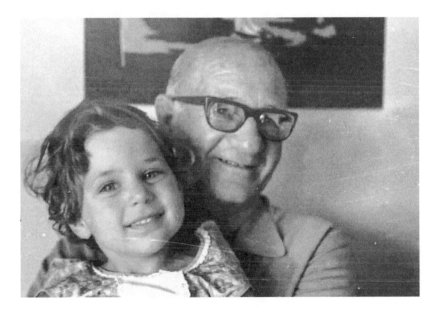

Contents

The Other
Family Doctor

1

It's a Calling

The cat had come with the house.

He was a feral black cat that John and Susan, who bought the tidy bungalow in a quiet tree-lined neighborhood, had named Miles. Many people wouldn't have concerned themselves with a stray, especially not when doing so cost them money. But although John and Susan hadn't expected Miles, they accepted him as their responsibility. They had him neutered and vaccinated at a nearby clinic. Miles warmed to his new humans, enjoying their attention even though he remained wild at heart, preferring to be outdoors most of the time. John and Susan allowed him into the house whenever he wanted, keeping him fed and warm. Slowly, he had become a part of their family.

But one chilly afternoon in February, John called me, his voice heavy with worry. He thought Miles might have an infected front paw. It was swollen, he explained over the phone, and Miles was limping. Suspecting an abscess, I told him it might need to be treated at a clinic. But as he and Susan were unable to catch Miles, I agreed to come to their house.

I was never happy about using a fishing net to catch a cat. I had learned the technique from another house-call veterinarian who specialized in cats and cared for some feral cat colonies. It always felt traumatic, especially when I knew the cats I cared for didn't understand. Still, I kept a fishing net in my car, if only to use as a last resort.

This was a last-resort kind of case.

When I arrived at their home, John and Susan led me to the back bathroom, where they'd been able to corral Miles. The poor kitty was petrified from being cooped up, and although he wouldn't allow me near him, I was able to trap him with the net. Wild creatures do not like being confined, and I hoped to be able to release him soon.

Remembering what the other vet had taught me, I used the double-wrapping method to enfold Miles until he was snug inside the net. My patient scratched and clawed, and I felt his distress. Yet I knew I had to be vigilant not to let him out or I wouldn't be able to catch him again. This was my one chance to help him. Finally, he settled and became still.

Biting my lip in concentration, I gently slid the long handle of the cat-net package a few feet along the linoleum floor into the kitchen, where the light was better and I had more room to work. I stood on the handle to hold the net in place. As soon as I looked closely at the paw, I could tell what was causing the limp. Occasionally a cat's claw will grow long enough to curl around in a circle and continue growing right into the pad, causing pain and often an infection. Miles had a badly ingrown nail, which had become embedded in his paw.

I would need to trim the nail to relieve Miles's pain and allow the infection to heal. However, I couldn't get to the nail with Miles compressed under the netting. Complicating matters, it was a front claw, close to Miles's sharp set of teeth. In a clinic setting, it would have taken two trained professionals using leather gloves to hold Miles so I could trim his nail safely, if it could be done at all. Otherwise, we'd have to anesthetize him. But here, hovering over Miles in the middle of the kitchen, none of those options was available to me.

I explained the problem to John and Susan and told them I didn't know what to do. They looked at me nervously. Although it would terrify Miles to go to a clinic, it would be a good option if I could get him into a carrier. But I doubted I'd be able to do that once I unwrapped him from the netting. And I had no injectable anesthetics with me, as that was not something I used in clients' homes. We had no good options.

As I stood there debating what to do next, this feral cat, trapped in the net, slowly extended the affected paw through the netting. The three of us watched, disbelieving, as he spread his toes. We looked at each other, mouths agape and soundless. That old thorn-in-the-lion's-paw story was flashing before our collective eyes.

As I quickly found my nail trimmers and cut the offending nail, Miles kept his paw completely still. None of us made a sound for fear of breaking whatever spell he was under. At last, I released Miles from the net. He shook himself and headed back outside. His limp was gone.

It was impossible to look at Miles, who would surely make a full recovery with the help of some antibiotics, and at John and Susan, who cared so much about this feral cat, and not think about the ways they had agreed to take care of each other and how, because of this, they were all better off.

I've been a veterinarian for thirty years. For most of that time I've had my own house-call practice, going inside people's homes to care for their animals, meeting my human clients and animal patients where they live. I've been in hundreds of residences, working at kitchen tables and living room sofas, even in bedrooms and bathrooms. Occasionally clients seem awkward as they invite me in, apologizing for clutter, dishes in a sink, or an unmade bed. "Don't worry at all," I respond. "No one sees *my* house!"

In this book, I am going to open my door and allow a view into my own home. You may see my clutter, my unmade bed, the dishes in my sink. You may witness how fully I've loved my own animals, and how I have struggled personally as well as professionally over the difficulties pet lovers face. And you can discover how much I have learned from my animal family members and patients about life, and love, and even death.

When people ask me when I knew I wanted to become a veterinarian, I tell them I've known my whole life. I have always loved animals. As a child, I drew them with crayons. I read books about them. I pretended to be a dog, a cat, or a horse and favored stuffed animals for toys. Yet one trip stands out in my memory as the moment when I knew I didn't just *want* to be a vet but *needed* to make animals a central part of my life.

Although I grew up in Massachusetts, my parents were born and raised in South Africa, and most of my extended family lived there. Holidays were lonely times for us because they highlighted what others had that we did not. While other people had family who visited them, who showered them with presents and hugs, we had only each other. We didn't have pets, either, as my mother said she had her hands full caring for myself and my brother. Then, however, came the opportunity to not only connect with my family but also to encounter the animals whose company I craved.

When I was a child, the fare for an international plane ticket was half price for children under twelve. My parents offered my younger brother, Michael, and me each a choice: at age eleven, we could either travel to South Africa to stay with family for the summer or we could save the money for a party to celebrate our bar or bat mitzvah when we turned thirteen. I immediately chose the trip.

I didn't know much about what to expect in Johannesburg when I arrived there in 1978, only that I would get to see my grandparents, aunts, uncles, cousins, and second cousins, many of them for the first time. I imagined what they would be like, these people who looked like me and spoke with accents like my parents'. I expected to finally get to see what their lives were like and to be spoiled by my grandparents. What I did not expect was that when I finally arrived, my aunt Hilary, uncle Leigh, and cousin Joanne would invite me on their weeklong safari vacation to Kruger National Park.

Kruger National Park is one of the largest game reserves in Africa. It has a land area roughly the size of Wales, and within its borders lives just about every kind of African animal imaginable: lions and zebras, elephants and giraffes, wildebeests and antelopes. The night before we left, I was so excited I could barely sleep. Little did I know this was one of those rare childhood moments when the excitement I felt beforehand paled in comparison to what it was like to experience the real thing.

On the appointed day, we piled into the family sedan, the car packed full of food and provisions, and, driving on what I thought was the wrong side of the road, headed north for several hours. As we drove, leaving behind the hustle and bustle of the city, Aunt Hilary explained the rules to me and four-year-old Joanne. "You can't get out of the car," she said. "Except when we are at the rest camp."

"What about bathrooms?" I asked.

"You go before we leave the camp. It's not safe to get out of the car. Sometimes it's not even safe *in* the car," she added. "I had a friend years ago whose car was trampled by an elephant. The parents had to jump into the back seat with the children. They were lucky they weren't killed."

This seemed impossible to me then, like a story adults told to scare children into compliance. Elephants could trample a car? What would that even look like? I was nervous but also thrilled at the idea of encountering creatures so big and powerful that they could crush our car to rubble. I longed to see them up close, to look into their eyes and see what kind of lives lived there.

Six hours felt like a very long time that day, as I constantly checked the clock to see how much longer we still had to go. We sang songs and played "I spy" until we were all sick of it. Eventually we drove through the gates of the park. Joanne and I positioned ourselves at the windows, spotting for wildlife.

"Look there!" said my uncle, pointing to a few impalas running across the road in front of us. The graceful antelopes leaped as though they were on springs. I didn't know yet that they were as common in the park as squirrels were at home. I was transfixed by their beauty and freedom. I watched them leap away in complete awe. But this was only the beginning.

We stayed at one of the many rest camps inside the park, where warthogs ran throughout like stray dogs as we walked around the grounds. Their large heads and long tusks made us giggle, as did the way they trotted along as though they were late to a meeting. In the morning, Aunt Hilary woke us when it was still dark outside. The animals, she explained, were most active at dusk and dawn; they slept through much of the day. We rubbed the sleep out of our eyes and piled into the sedan.

As we drove through the long, straight roads of the park, the African sun painting the sky a deep orange, we were enraptured. We saw zebras, elephants, and giraffes. Hippos. Baboons. An elegant kudu, a type of antelope with large curling horns. Silly-looking wildebeests, also called gnus. Large herds of impalas, graceful and leaping. Occasionally, vultures circled overhead. It was winter in the southern hemisphere, and the limited vegetation made it easier to see the wildlife. I took pictures with my little Kodak Instamatic camera, hoping the photos would provide proof of the amazing sights I was experiencing, as well as memories I could hold on to when I eventually had to go back home.

Some animals were common, like the impalas; others were rarer, like lions. Each time we spotted one, we stopped to watch. We could drive for hours without seeing another car, but when we did notice a stopped car ahead, it elicited great excitement. *What did they spot?* we wondered. *A pride of lions? A rhino? Hyenas?* Each time, I felt like the lucky winner of an out-of-body experience, able to encounter the world through the eyes of something wild.

One day a swarm of monkeys enveloped our car. They were on the roof, on the hood, on the ground. My cousin and I pointed at a mother carrying a baby monkey. "So cute!"

"Don't open the windows!" my uncle shouted. We guessed that some people had fed the monkeys through car windows and now they were looking for food. I didn't open my window, but I held up my hands to the glass as I met a monkey's eyes. I wished I could touch him.

In the distance, we at last spotted what we had been hoping to see. It was a herd of elephants. They were enormous, bigger than I had imagined, like houses come to life. As soon as we saw them, Aunt Hilary, who was driving, turned the car around while keeping a respectful distance, explaining, "If they charge, I want to be able to drive forward, not in reverse." I was impressed that she could keep her wits about her in that moment when all I could manage to do was gawk. The large figures were so improbable, they looked as though they'd been created by Dr. Seuss. I wanted to get out of the car and stand close to them, but I knew that was impossible. Although the animals had become accustomed to the cars driving around and mostly ignored them, a person outside a vehicle could easily be viewed as prey, and you never knew what dangerous animal might be lurking nearby. I also knew that although the elephants looked slow-moving, they could move fast when they wanted to. We didn't want to anger them. This was their world, and we were the lucky visitors, compelled to obey their rules.

All too soon, our trip was coming to an end. I was trying to soak up every last bit of wildlife I could, sure that if I could just bottle up these memories, I could hold on to them for the rest of my life. I don't remember where we were driving or what we had just seen when, without warning, we happened upon a tree with a half-eaten impala carcass slung across a high fork of branches. Its head and front legs were dangling limply toward the ground. All four of us collectively gasped.

We could only guess that a predator, likely one of the big cats, had carried it up into the tree for safekeeping until the hunter was ready to eat again. I thought my aunt and uncle would quickly drive past it, but instead they lingered. Years later, I wondered what this had taught me, even if I didn't recognize it at the time: about the fierce nature of the animal kingdom; about the way that life always exists in concert with death, not in opposition to it; that to love animals, to care for them, means recognizing that they will always die.

But this was not the only lesson I would learn as a result of that trip. As we watched the animals in their natural habitats, I was struck by the knowledge that they had been living so peacefully without humans. I kept wondering, what can we learn from them? What can they teach us? These animals looked odd when viewed as pictures or inside zoos. But they appeared far more sensible in their own environments. The long neck of a giraffe, stretched to nibble leaves on the top of a tree, did not look funny. It seemed perfectly natural. Confined to our cars, we were the ones who seemed out of place. It was my first lesson in the importance of context when considering an animal's well-being.

But animals were not the only ones to help me with that understanding. My first teacher, who helped me learn the necessity of what would later be termed narrative medicine, was in fact my grandfather.

My grandfather Maurice Fine was a physician in South Africa. My brother and I called him Oupa (pronounced *oh-pah*), which means "grandfather" in the Afrikaans language. He was short, balding, and usually smiling. Oupa was an old-style type of doctor, a general practitioner. He treated the entire family, adults and children alike. He delivered babies and cared for the elderly. A soft-spoken, patient man, he took his time and gave each person his focused attention. Oupa maintained a small office where he saw patients, but he also made house calls, which accounted for about half of his practice.

When I was a child, my grandparents came to America almost every summer to visit us, so I got to know them well. Oupa loved to sing, and you could often tell where he was in the house by the sound of him singing or humming old show tunes or lighthearted melodies, like "It's a Long Way to Tipperary" and "The Ugly Duckling." I still remember the way my grandfather applied a Band-Aid (or a plaster, as he called it): slowly and carefully, placing the soft cotton part over the skin before pulling off the tabs. The first thing he did if I approached him with a medical problem, whether a headache or a scraped knee, was to take my pulse with his gentle hands. As he held my small hand between his two, I felt calmed.

In my grandfather's day, doctors were respected, but not placed on a pedestal. Oupa was a member of his community, one who drove from home to home doing his rounds, checking in on his patients. He bartered with some of them, taking care of the family of a local mechanic who in turn cared for my grandfather's car for many years. Neither kept track; they considered it an even trade.

"How can you take care of a patient if you've never been to their home?" he'd wonder aloud. I knew this wasn't really a question.

In their homes, Oupa could tell which of his patients were taking their medications, who had a healthy lifestyle, and who was a chronic smoker even though they denied it. If he noticed drawn curtains on a sunny day or a messy home that used to be tidy, he might suspect a patient was depressed, which informed his treatment plan. When someone came to his office, he already knew them well from having been in their home.

My grandfather's lifestyle sounded idyllic to me, except for the fact that he lived and practiced in South Africa under apartheid. My parents had explained apartheid to my brother and me, as much as the government-mandated racial separation policy could be explained. My family was fairly new to South Africa, as my great-grandparents were a part of the Jewish population that settled there after fleeing persecution in Russia around the turn of the century.

The ideals of my grandparents were not in line with those of the South African government. Eventually, two of their three children left the authoritarian country and emigrated to England, then America. My father's sister, Hazel, and her husband, Hymie, left before my parents; they were active in the anti-apartheid movement and, although I didn't know it at the time, they had once hidden Nelson Mandela in their home for several weeks when he was evading police. When my aunt and uncle received word that the authorities were asking questions about them, they had to flee the country within hours. They lived in exile, unable to return for over twenty years, fearing arrest.

My grandparents would likely have emigrated as well, but their third child was severely disabled, and they would not have been able to afford his care had they moved. So they settled for annual visits and aerograms, the light blue, prestamped, paper and envelope in one, which were the main form of communication between separated families in those days. Phone calls back then were prohibitively expensive and reserved for emergencies. It was always hard saying goodbye at the end of my grandparents' summer visit, knowing I wouldn't see them or hear their voices for another whole year, other than a birthday phone call lasting only a couple of minutes.

When I left South Africa that summer, I was sad to be departing but excited to get home to my bird, Taffy. For my eleventh birthday, the fall before my South Africa trip, my mother had allowed me to get a parakeet. It was the family's first pet. My father brought me to the local Woolworth's, where I had picked out a bright green budgie. I was ecstatic to have a pet of my own, right there in my room. I watched her in awe, this beautiful tiny creature, hopping around in her cage. I had purchased a book on parakeets, which I read from cover to cover. I wanted to do everything I could to keep my bird happy. Taffy had mirrors and toys in her cage, even sandpaper covers for her perches to prevent her nails from growing too long.

I hoped to have Taffy jump on my finger, but she was nervous and easily frightened. I, however, possessed the patience and the determination of an extreme animal lover with her first pet, and the free time of an eleven-year-old in the 1970s. I stood in front of her cage for hours at a time, every day, with the door open and my index finger barely inside, waiting for Taffy to adjust to my presence. I held my finger straight out like a perch and moved it in the tiniest possible increments so she wouldn't jump away. Eventually, I got close to her as she sat on her favorite perch by the mirror.

One day, I managed to gently touch my finger to her chest. Then Taffy surprised me by climbing onto the extended digit, one little bird foot at a time, gripping tightly to maintain her balance on the unfamiliar perch. I stood still, elated. It was one of the happiest moments of my life.

That day proved to be a turning point; I had won Taffy's trust, and she and I were inseparable from then on. She hopped willingly onto my finger every day when I got home from school and went anywhere in the house with me. I began leaving her cage door open when I was in the room with her, so she could fly around. She sang to me, and I sang back to her.

When my mother started working full-time, a problem arose. We wanted to turn the heat down during the day, but parakeets require a warm temperature. My father created a special, large cage for Taffy with a thermostat and a light bulb for a heat source. We kept her cage in the kitchen.

One day when I was in high school, I came home from school and went into the kitchen for a snack. My eyes couldn't find Taffy on any of her perches; she was on her back, on the bottom of the cage, dead. I ran out of the room, screaming, and called my father at work. He buried her that evening, under a small pine tree we could see from the kitchen window. She had loved to look out that window, perched on the wide edge of a clay mug my brother had made, and I often looked up at her on the windowsill as I waited for the school bus. Taffy's death took me completely by surprise, as she had shown no signs of illness before she died. It was three days before I could bring myself to venture into the kitchen again. I felt as though it was the end of my childhood.

My grief for Taffy was no less than it would have been for a dog or a cat. Yes, I was still a child, and she was only a little bird. But grief over the loss of a dear friend is the same no matter what your age, and no matter what the species.

Just as I couldn't imagine Oupa doing anything else other than being a doctor, I couldn't imagine wanting to be anything except a veterinarian, especially after that trip of a lifetime where I felt connected to the animals around me in a new, deeper way. I wanted to take care of them the same way my grandfather took care of people: learning their stories, connecting with them, and making them feel safe. For both of us, being a doctor was a calling. It was as simple and as mystifying as that.

I knew that becoming a veterinarian would require many years of schooling, but I did well in school and was prepared to do whatever was necessary to follow my dream. Also, my parents had always stressed the importance of education. One day, my father explained why.

"It's because we're Jewish. Our people have been forced to move countries many times. If you put your money into education, that's something you can bring with you, and it can't be stolen. It's safer than putting it in a bank."

It was a solemn reminder of my family's history.

Soon, however, an unexpected obstacle to my chosen career arose: allergies. In high school, I volunteered at a local veterinary clinic, where I sneezed uncontrollably whenever a cat entered the room. Eventually, I stopped being present for feline exams and treatment.

"Don't even think about going to veterinary school," my allergist told me. Sitting across from him in his office, I crossed my arms and frowned. Maybe I just wouldn't treat cats, I decided. Of course I was still going to go to veterinary school—if I managed to get accepted, that is. I resolved to find a way to make it work, even if it meant sneezing every day for the rest of my life. Caring for animals was that important to me.

I already knew veterinary school was notoriously hard to get into, due in part to the limited number of schools. If I had been born one or more decades earlier, I would have had another barrier: being a woman.

Several women older than me have told me that many veterinary schools refused to admit women. Even when women began to be consistently accepted to veterinary schools, about ten years before me, they did not have it easy. "You realize you're taking away a spot from a man?" a friend was asked. The implication was that men needed to support families and women did not, and that men were stronger and therefore more physically capable of treating animals. While, admittedly, most women are smaller physically than most men, when faced with a horse or a cow, a hundred pounds doesn't make a lot of difference.

I chose an undergraduate university with a strong premed department, as veterinary schools require the completion of most of the same courses as medical schools in order to apply. At Brandeis University, I took biology, chemistry, organic chemistry, and physics, all with lab courses, in addition to regular classes. It was a rigorous curriculum, and premed students were advised to not play sports or apply to junior-year study-abroad programs if they wanted to succeed. Although I enjoyed my college biology class, organic chemistry and physics did not come naturally to me. Looking back, I wonder at them being requirements. Many doctors I know have speculated that prerequisite science courses existed more to weed out students than anything else. In practice, I've never used physics or organic chemistry. However, two subjects that were not required are ones I use regularly, even daily: psychology and ethics. Much of psychology is applicable to both humans and animals (Pavlov, after all, used dogs in his studies). And I often find myself in situations with complex ethics involving both my animal patient and human client.

During vacations, I worked as a receptionist at a local veterinary clinic. I wasn't working directly with cats, so my allergies were not a problem. Although I didn't get to see the animals up close, I was learning how to talk to clients about their pets' problems. As the reception desk overlooked the waiting room, I often heard people exchange anecdotes about their animals. One day a man yelled at me, irate that he had to wait for his dog's appointment instead of being allowed to drop off his pet. After sitting in the waiting room and exchanging animal stories with other pet owners for about half an hour, he calmed down so much that he apologized before he left. It was my first indication that being a vet wouldn't just involve caring for animals, but, in many ways, for their owners, too.

The clinic was also my first real glimpse of the inner workings of an animal hospital. The receptionists served as the gatekeepers: booking appointments, fielding questions from clients on the phone, and checking clients in and out. The technician staff acted as nurses and assistants. They worked with the doctors in the exam room or in surgery, ran tests in the lab area of the facility, or directly provided patient care. Veterinarians saw clients or performed surgery. And an office manager was the one who had hired me and oversaw the whole operation.

I enjoyed watching the doctors talk to clients and observing lab work and surgeries when I had the chance. One dog, named Split for her tendency to lie with her front legs spread apart, had difficulty recovering from an emergency splenectomy and spent the following few days lying down in her run. We all worried about her, and the entire staff cheered when she rallied and stood for the first time. I had never participated in organized sports, but I imagined that this was how it felt when your team scores the winning point.

Occasionally, my father would ask if I wanted to apply to medical school instead of veterinary school. Both require an elaborate screening process with numerous entrance requirements. Both have a great deal of competition for available spots. Both consist of four years of rigorous study following four years of undergraduate college. Students in both schools learn anatomy, physiology, and the recognition, treatment, and prevention of disease processes. The main difference is while physicians learn to treat only humans, veterinarians must learn to practice on more than one species. Other differences include veterinarians' ability to enter general practice without having to specialize and complete a residency. And, of course, the reality that veterinarians earn far less money than physicians was not lost on my father.

I knew all this. Yet I told him that I had no desire to be a medical doctor. I didn't want to become a vet for the money. I would argue that none of us do.

The fall of my senior year of college, it was time to mail my veterinary school application to Tufts. Tufts was the only veterinary school in New England, so I was most likely to be admitted there, since students were accepted based on geographical location. I tried to remain undaunted when a midwestern veterinary school declined to send me an application, informing me that my preliminary transcript did not meet their minimum requirements.

At the main post office in town, I climbed the steps of the brick building with my paperwork painstakingly assembled in a large manila envelope. It felt enormously important, this day I had worked toward for what seemed my entire life. I knew that many people applied for years before getting accepted to veterinary school, and many others were wait-listed, but I was hopeful. My grades were steady, and I had volunteered at the veterinary school and done well on the required GRE test, obtaining a near-perfect score on the logic portion. On the other hand, Tufts had not accepted me into their undergraduate program.

The odds of admission were slim; today they hover at around 11 percent. Several weeks later, I was encouraged when I received a letter with the news that I had been granted an interview, which I knew increased my chances. On the big day, I sat in a chair in the hallway of the large brick admissions building awaiting my turn, wearing uncomfortable interview clothing and taking deep breaths. When I was finally called, the two interviewers were friendly but showed no reaction as I answered their questions. I felt good about some of my answers, and concerned about others, but their expressions didn't change, so I had no idea what they thought. I went home and cried. All I could do now was wait.

Months later, I stood in front of my student mailbox, holding a letter bearing the blue Tufts seal in the upper left-hand corner. It felt thick, a good sign. I opened the envelope and read the words I'd been hoping to see. I felt as though I were floating, like all the pieces of my life had come together for this moment to arrive.

I had been accepted.

What I didn't realize then, having been focused for so long on *getting into* veterinary school, was how hard it would be to *stay* in veterinary school. Now the real work would have to begin. I would learn to be a veterinarian, to live a life surrounded by animals, and to help them the way that my grandfather helped his patients— by learning their stories and, slowly over time, becoming a part of them. Even in ways I couldn't have anticipated.

2

Veterinary School

In preparation for veterinary school, I rented an apartment just outside Boston with one of my future classmates, a woman from New Jersey named Wendy. Wendy was a good choice for a roommate as she was easy to get along with, already had living room furniture (I did not), and was a good cook (my repertoire consisted of macaroni and cheese from a box and chocolate chip cookies from scratch).

Wendy also had a cat. Fortunately I seemed to have outgrown my sneezing allergy to cats, or I built up a tolerance to them while working at the clinic in college. For the first time in my life, I realized, I could have a cat of my own.

I knew just where I wanted to go to adopt one: a shelter called Buddy Dog. I was familiar with the shelter because during college I had participated in a volunteer program that involved bringing animals to visit a nearby nursing home once a month.

Each visit began at the shelter, where a staff member helped me choose a friendly puppy, kitten, or both, depending on which animals were available that day. I then drove to a nursing home about thirty minutes away and spent a pleasant hour or so with the residents. I watched as faces lit up, eyes softened, and hands reached out to touch the animals. I listened as people told stories of animals they'd known and loved. Many talked about childhood pets, animals who had died decades ago. One woman always asked if the puppy and the kitten were brother and sister; I never knew if she was asking if they belonged to the same family or whether she thought they were actually related. My answer was always a cheerful "No, they're not." More than once, at the end of the visit, a tearful staff member approached me to confide that a resident who'd been animated and talkative with the animals present hadn't spoken or interacted with anyone for days beforehand. I was pleased but not surprised; I understood what animals could do for people.

This time, I headed toward Buddy Dog to choose an animal to keep. In the kitten room, tiny paws stretched through metal cage bars as I walked back and forth. I didn't have a color or gender in mind. In one cage, I spotted a gray-striped tiger kitten with iridescent green eyes. When I took him out of the cage, he clung to me as if he knew we belonged together. I trusted him immediately.

I named him Daiquiri because I loved how the word sounds. He got along well with Wendy's older kitten, Kali, and they played and napped together. He slept on my bed each night and finished the last spoonful of milk from my cereal every morning (while some cats are lactose intolerant, Dai had no problems with his dairy treat).

My college boyfriend of three years was starting medical school about an hour away. We'd nearly broken up the previous year, and although I went to visit him in his new apartment, he seemed to want to keep me separate from his medical school life. When my boyfriend finally visited me, he wasn't happy that I'd gotten a cat. He said he was allergic (something I didn't recall him ever mentioning)—but seemed more jealous than anything else. "How do you know the cat loves you?" he asked. "Maybe he just likes you because you feed him." Not long afterward, we broke up.

It was easier this way, I realized. The relationship had been plagued by ups and downs, and was often draining. Now I could really focus on my studies. Once I got over the initial devastation of the breakup, I welcomed being single.

During my early twenties, as my working friends enjoyed themselves on weeknights, went out on weekends, and even dated, my classmates and I studied almost constantly. Veterinary school consisted of full days of classes and labs, and each evening involved several hours of studying. Weekends meant laundry and grocery shopping, as well as more time to study. The vast amounts of material presented seemed impossible to master, no matter how many hours I worked.

There was also the commute to adjust to, as Wendy and I had to travel from our apartment in Somerville to the Tufts medical school campus in downtown Boston each day. As the veterinary school campus could not yet accommodate everyone, first- and second-year veterinary students were crammed into a couple of windowless basement rooms in the medical school building thirty miles from the rural veterinary campus. Wendy and I took a bus to the T station, rode the train several stops, then walked a few more blocks to school. For months at a time, the only animals I saw other than the ones I lived with were rats scurrying around in the subway.

The first week of school, I became friendly with another student named Karen. We ate lunch together, along with an assortment of other classmates. One weekend, we arranged to study together at the medical school library. We organized ourselves at nearby study carrels and read our syllabi, breaking every hour or so to chat. At one point, Karen became overwhelmed by the amount of material we had to cover. As I tried to cheer her up, I had a flash of inspiration. I retrieved my Walkman (or Walkperson, as I called it) from my backpack and checked the tape inside. Yep, Bob Marley. I rewound to the song "No Woman No Cry," which repeats the phrase *everything's gonna be all right* so many times that you begin to believe it.

"This will help," I promised Karen as I handed her the head-phones. She adjusted them, leaned back, closed her eyes, and started to sway ever so slightly as her body relaxed and she began to smile. After the song, she was herself again.

"Hey, how 'bout we go to Chinatown for lunch after we finish the next section?" she asked. "I know some really good places that aren't too expensive." Karen knew Chinatown well, and we enjoyed a delicious meal as she taught me how to use chopsticks.

During another study session, I asked Karen a question. "How late are you up on Saturday nights, usually?" I had agreed to have dinner with my ex-boyfriend the following weekend, something that had seemed like a good idea when he'd called. Now I wasn't so sure. I didn't exactly want to cancel, but I knew Karen was a night owl and I thought maybe I could talk to her when I got home if things went badly.

"You can call me *anytime*," she responded firmly after I explained. She put her hand on my arm for emphasis. "Just remember, I can be at your place in twenty minutes with a bottle of wine." Those words remain one of the finest declarations of friendship I have ever heard.

Most weeks, our entire class was together for thirty to forty hours, so we got to know one another well. If someone got a new sweater, we all noticed. Most time was spent in the dark, watching slide presentations from various professors. I sometimes resorted to eating to try to stay awake and lined up my water bottle and a granola bar and whatever else I had brought. Notes in the form of small folded papers were surreptitiously passed from row to row and seat to seat for communication. *Staying late to study today? Did you finish the chapter? Want to eat lunch outside?* Outside meant the steps of the church next door, a sunny spot we sometimes shared with homeless people.

Most of our teachers were men, but my class was on the cusp of a large change in the profession: we were 70 percent female, a record. Tufts never had a policy of excluding women, and women were beginning to apply to veterinary schools in record numbers. The trend has continued, as more women than men graduate from veterinary schools today. A likely reason is that more men choose to enter human medicine due to the far-higher pay in that field for approximately the same years of study and costs in student loans.

We heard that the class two years ahead of us included some female students who had complained loudly about sexist remarks from various professors, resulting in the administration instituting policies to decrease such comments.

"At this point in the lecture, there's a joke I like to tell, but now, you know, I've been told I'm not *supposed* to," a professor might complain, eliciting cries of "Tell! Tell!" from a few classmates, as I silently thanked those who came before me.

I commiserated with my college friend Maddy, who was in medical school in Maryland. Maddy's class was a record 50 percent women. "You know how professors like to throw in a fun slide at the beginning or end of the lecture?" she asked me. "Well, some of my professors show a scantily clad woman." I was appalled. All my professors, without exception, either showed slides of their own pets or *Far Side* cartoons for their "fun slides."

In theory, one of the reasons the first two years of our veterinary classes were located on the medical school campus was to share some of their faculty, and we had a few physiology lectures together with the medical students. My classmates and I heard rumors about a tradition of some medical students sitting in the back row to make mooing sounds, which sounded comical to me. The rumor turned out to be true, but when I was in the classroom and actually heard the moos, I was not amused. It seemed condescending and disrespectful. Was this really how physicians viewed veterinarians?

The medical school and veterinary school anatomy labs were side by side, in the basement of an old building across the street from our classroom building. My fellow veterinary students and I spent what seemed like countless hours in those basement rooms, feeling pickled ourselves from the formaldehyde fumes, dissecting our cadaver dogs (and later, ponies) in student groups of three. We took turns reading from the anatomy book and dissecting with the metal instruments. Occasionally, a handful of medical students would drift down the hallway and stand in the doorway to peer into our room.

"*Ewww*, you do dogs?"

Some of us returned the favor, slipping away from our lab to gaze curiously into the medical school anatomy room. "Wow, people. *Ewww*."

And it did seem strange to see, there on the familiar metal table, a form so akin to my own. Otherwise, the medical student lab was nearly identical to ours: the bright lights, the pungent smell of formaldehyde, the heads of classmates bent together over books and bodies. I was friendly with some medical students, and they invited us in for a closer look. My lab partners and I examined a human cadaver up close. Looking under the skin, we saw that the muscles, blood vessels, organs, and tissues appeared much the same as those we were dissecting in our neighboring room.

Exams were grueling, and typically consisted of page after page of multiple-choice questions featuring treacherous combinations such as "A and C," "none of the above," or "all of the above." My classmates each had their own ritual for pre-exam nerves. In the hallway and the break room before an exam, we resembled Olympic athletes anxiously waiting to compete; like them, we had practiced and sacrificed and now had one chance to demonstrate our abilities and be judged accordingly. Some students huddled in small groups, comparing how little sleep they'd had and which sections they'd struggled with most. Others frantically paged through textbooks, syllabi, or homemade index cards while mumbling to themselves.

I chose neither option. To center myself, I tried to connect with the reason I was there in the first place. I always had my Walkperson with me, as music helped me relax and focus. During my commute I listened to the Indigo Girls, Suzanne Vega, Tracy Chapman, UB40, and many others, but there was one tape reserved for exams: U2's *The Joshua Tree*. I sat (or possibly curled into the fetal position) on the sofa in the break room with my headphones on and my eyes closed. I related to the passion in the music; it felt so close to my deep desire of wanting to become a veterinarian.

After a final exam, on, say, a Wednesday night in December, a random group of us might celebrate, going out for lunch in Chinatown or, later, heading to a bar or a nightclub and dancing until the wee hours. We'd split an order of nachos, as they were cheap and filling, and we favored a bar near school that offered ninety-nine-cent drafts. Those times were rare, but they helped bond us together, myself and my seventy or so classmates.

My class was only the veterinary school's tenth, and it is a testament to the teachers and the school administration that our education did not feel scattered despite the split campus. Our teachers were knowledgeable and often intense, devoted to both our education and their fields. Sometimes we had a sense that they argued over the amount of time allotted to their individual fields; the cardiologists wanted to give us more lectures, as did most of the other specialties.

I didn't realize until years later that functioning under less-than-ideal circumstances has long been a hallmark of veterinary medicine. Veterinarians have a history of making do, utilizing old equipment salvaged from human hospitals like anesthesia and X-ray machines. Only recently have such devices been widely marketed for the purposes of veterinary medicine. Veterinarians excel at using what they have on hand; for instance, fashioning a splint for a kitten from a tongue depressor. My profession is filled with outside-the-box thinkers who persist until they find a way to make something work.

I was interested in working internationally, and I knew I needed more large-animal experience. After my first year, I found a summer job living and working on a dairy farm in Upstate New York. It was a different lifestyle than I had ever experienced growing up in the suburbs of Boston. Everything revolved around the farm animals and their needs. I saw firsthand the meaning of expressions such as *make hay while the sun shines* and *until the cows come home*. I learned how to drive a tractor, and the farmer, Doug, gifted me a baby goat.

It was a far cry from my fourth-floor apartment in Somerville. When I tried to explain where I lived to Doug, I could tell it was hard for him to comprehend life in the city. He and his wife, Carol, owned the land they lived on and farmed. "If I get up at night and go for a walk in my sleep, I need to know that I'd be on my own land," he told me. I struggled to relate.

Doug's favorite treat was a visit to a local diner called the Bluebird for a slice of pie. He referred to the restaurant as the "Dirty Bird," more out of a sense of familiarity than disrespect. The town was small and everyone seemed to know each other. Once, as we sat at the diner counter, a regular asked the waitress for a glass of milk. "Okay, but finish your water first so I don't have to dirty another glass," she responded. I nearly spat out my pie.

I didn't realize how I had romanticized the life of a farmer—

living in harmony with the land and the animals—until something happened one day in the barn. I'd heard Doug complain about swallows nesting there but hadn't thought much of it until I saw him take a broom handle and aim it into the rafters. Too late, I realized what was going on. He'd knocked down a swallow's nest with just-hatched eggs, which had fallen directly into the back of the manure spreader, a large trailer filled with manure that Doug or I would tow with the tractor to fertilize the hay fields.

I didn't hesitate, scrambling on top of the pile of droppings, searching for baby birds. I found them, featherless and new, covered in manure. It was too late, I could tell. They would not survive.

I ran back to the house in tears, ignoring Doug's appeals to me. He had no idea why I was so upset. He had nothing against swallows; he just didn't like bird poop in the barn. On the farm, the worth of an animal corresponded to its ability to contribute economically to the entire system. Even though they were beautiful to watch, if the birds created more work, then their lives held no value. It was a hard thing for me to comprehend, and it was a couple of days before I stopped picturing those doomed baby birds covered in manure and was able to forgive Doug.

One day a little while after the swallow incident, I walked into the barn. It must have been milking time—it seemed as though it was always milking time there on the farm: twice a day, every day. On that day, the cows had been brought in from the fields and were in their stalls, waiting for the farmer and me to attach the milking machines to each cow in turn.

As I walked down the center aisle, cow tails swishing away on both sides of me, I noticed one cow lying down, lazily munching some hay. She didn't see me approach until I was almost directly behind her, at which point, she startled and jumped. Her entire black-and-white Holstein body, likely about fifteen hundred pounds, gave an enormous spasm as she turned her head and looked at me, wide-eyed. It was such a human thing to do; I could picture her thinking, *Where the heck did you come from? You* scared *me!* The cow did not possess human speech, but she communicated with me through her body language and her eyes. I related to her experience the same way I would have if I'd seen or read about a person being startled, or watched it on TV. As I had clearly witnessed, being startled is not solely a human phenomenon. It made me wonder about the concept of anthropomorphizing—attributing human emotions and responses to animals. Animals, I suspected, possess far more similarities to us than differences, and many more abilities than we give them credit for. Why should we assume that humans are the gold standard of experience and emotions, for other species to be measured against?

Back in Boston, second year began; we were done with anatomy and had learned much of the medical vocabulary and terminology we needed to communicate. However, the pace did not diminish. Classes now focused on problems affecting different body systems such as the gastrointestinal (GI) tract and the heart, as well as pharmacology and parasitology.

After receiving a D on an exam one fall day, I skipped class, something rare for me. I just couldn't face another hour in the dark basement room, especially feeling sad and disappointed. It was a nice day, and I walked over to Downtown Crossing by the famous Filene's Basement. I people-watched, listened to the sparrows chirp, and splurged on a warm scarf from one of the pushcart vendors. I didn't think of it as self-care, but it helped. I returned ready to work even harder.

Soon I had something exciting to focus on. My father was going on a business trip to South Africa and had enough frequent-flier miles to bring me with him. We planned the trip to coincide with my spring break in March. I was thrilled to think of spending time with family I hadn't seen since my last trip nearly seven years earlier. I would see my grandparents, as well as my aunt Hilary and her family. I could meet my three-year-old cousin Brad for the first time and see my aunt Joy and uncle Chris. I would miss seeing my aunt Sue, uncle Don, and young cousin Janine, as they had recently immigrated to Australia.

As usual, there were also the conflicting feelings of visiting people I loved, but in a country with a racist system of government. However, change was afoot. Although apartheid was still in place, Nelson Mandela had just been released from jail after being held as a political prisoner for twenty-seven years. I had jumped for joy at the news. I was in awe of his leadership ability after such a long prison sentence; I was convinced I wouldn't know my own name after so many years imprisoned, yet he had held fast to his ideals. South Africans were hopeful for a peaceful end to the authoritarian system, and there was talk of a "new" South Africa. But first, all citizens would need the right to vote, which was still restricted to the white minority.

I'd been meeting with my faculty adviser, Chip, to plan an international trip for the summer. I had received grant money to conduct a project with a veterinarian who was working in the Peace Corps in Morocco. When I told Chip about my upcoming South Africa trip, he had an interesting offer. Another student a couple of years ahead of me had been trying to start a student exchange program with MEDUNSA, the Black veterinary school in South Africa. MEDUNSA stood for Medical University of South Africa. The white veterinary school, Onderstepoort, was a full-fledged, internationally known institution. The apartheid laws mandated racially separate educational facilities, with the Black facilities receiving far less money and resources. MEDUNSA was near Johannesburg, and if I could visit the school in person and meet with the students, it could help make progress on the student exchange program idea. I was excited to help in any way I could. I felt guilty about visiting family there and supporting apartheid in that way; here was something I could do to make up for a small portion of it.

I had last visited South Africa during high school for a family wedding. Then, we'd been able to travel directly from the United States, a long-haul flight of around sixteen hours. Since then, the United States had instituted sanctions against the South African government in protest of apartheid, and direct flights were no longer allowed between the two countries. Travelers from the United States typically flew through Europe. My father was already going to be in London for a meeting, so I would meet him there and we would fly together to Johannesburg.

Several family members met us at the airport, including my grandparents and Aunt Hilary. It felt good to be welcomed so warmly after such a long journey. South Africa had never been my home, but it felt like home in some ways. Staying with family was comfortable and familiar. I had favorite foods: South African candy bars, dried biscuits called rusks, and the giant Indian samosas (pronounced *sa-MOO-sas*). I listened to South African music by Ladysmith Black Mambazo, Hugh Masekela, and Miriam Makeba. Hilary brought me to outdoor marketplaces where I learned how to barter and bought beaded jewelry.

In Johannesburg, my parents' accents were the norm instead of the exception. Sometimes I heard my parents use an expression that wasn't "American English," and I didn't know whether it was an African thing, a Jewish thing, or just unique to my family. "I'll do it *just-now*" was something my father often said when he meant "I'll do it soon." "I'll do it *this-now*" was often said with irritation and clearly meant "I'll do it later, and stop asking me." These different ways of referring to time turned out to be a South African thing, and I heard other people use the expressions while I was there. In

South Africa, things I didn't understand at home seemed to click and make sense.

One morning, my father woke me early and we headed to the airport for a flight to Cape Town. I was going to meet my father's brother for the first time. In Cape Town, we rented a car for the two-hour drive to the small town of Swellendam, where my uncle Ray lived.

My father, at the age of eight, had contracted mumps. At the time, there was no vaccine against the disease. He recovered uneventfully, but his four-year-old brother, Ray, also got sick. As a complication of the virus, Ray developed encephalitis, an inflammation of the brain. He survived, but his brain was irreparably damaged. For the rest of his life, Ray had the intellectual capacity of a two-year-old child. He could speak a few words, but it was difficult for him to communicate, and when frustrated he sometimes turned to the tantrums two-year-olds are known for. The only thing that seemed to help was music. Oupa sang to him, and my uncle, who could not put together a full sentence on his own, had memorized dozens of songs and would sing along, calming down and focusing on the music. However, as a six-foot young adult, Ray was difficult for my grandparents to control, and it was hard to get him to do anything he didn't want to do. Oupa's friend Adriaan offered a solution: he ran a boarding school in a small town outside Cape Town. Ray could live in a little cottage on the premises with a caretaker. He would be a part of the community. Adriaan's suggestion worked out well, and Ray had lived there since the early 1970s.

When we arrived, I recognized Ray from photos I had seen. He looked a little like Oupa, but taller. My uncle was thrilled to see my father and bellowed, "DA-vid! DA-vid!" over and over. My father tried to explain that I was his daughter, and Ray's niece, but my uncle did not understand, so he ignored me. We brought Ray for a drive, his favorite activity, preferably ending with an ice cream. As I sat in the back seat behind my father, Ray continued to repeat my father's name and began thumping him heartily on the back. My father, several inches shorter than his brother, flinched and put up his arm to protect himself. "Not while I'm driving, Ray, not while I'm driving!" he yelled. "Let's sing, okay? What shall we sing?" Soon they were singing, and Ray calmed down.

I knew my father well, but I had never seen him with his brother. Ray had been almost a mythical figure to me. His illness had dramatically changed his life as well as the lives of my grandparents, my father, and my aunt Hazel. I imagined how difficult it must have been for Oupa, as a doctor as well as a parent, for his own child to have a devastating illness he was unable to treat; how bittersweet the eventual release of the vaccination for mumps, too late for Ray, but enabling Oupa to prevent the disease in his patients. My grandfather never spoke about these things; he appeared happy to live in the present.

After a couple of days with Ray, we drove back to Cape Town and my father showed me the crashing waves of Muizenberg Beach, which he'd visited as a child with his family. Unable to stay at a hotel because Ray was disruptive, they had rented a house in an area called Fish Hoek. My father recalled that he sometimes tanned so dark during beach vacations that the local deli owner refused to serve him, sending him out of the shop. At the time, my father had been amused. It was before the watershed moment that changed his view of race forever, which had happened back in Johannesburg. In the car, my father told me the story.

"When I was a teenager, I was coming home from school and saw a Black man who was bleeding, staggering up the street in search of our house to find my father, the doctor. I remember seeing the wound and the blood coming from it, and I was surprised by the fact that a Black man had red blood just like me. I was shaken to the core as the realization hit me as to what apartheid was all about. It was an awful shock to realize just how manipulated we all were, even growing up with a very liberal and forward-thinking father and a large extended family, some of whom were also liberal in outlook. I decided then and there that I had to find a way to either change this madness or to escape from it. I vowed to never build a life on the backs of other people."

I had heard this story before, but never in the country where it had happened. It always amazed me that my father, the most ethical, wise, and generous person I knew, could have held such a belief. He always thought things through, considered every angle, and tried to be a good person. I'd been shocked one day to see him eat a grape in the supermarket while we were grocery shopping. It was horrifying to hear about the racism that had seeped into him as a child without his knowledge or consent.

A couple of days after we arrived back in Johannesburg, my father and I set off for MEDUNSA. After years of driving on the right side of the road in the United States, my father found it difficult to adjust to driving on the left again, especially on unfamiliar roads. Each time we approached an intersection, he repeated out loud, "The driver's in the middle of the road. The driver's in the middle of the road," to remind himself not to revert to right-side driving. It made the trip a bit nerve-racking. Fortunately, as we neared MEDUNSA, the intersections became fewer, as the school was in a rural area.

At the campus, we met with the hospital director as well as the dean of the school. A student named Langa, the chairperson of the veterinary students, gave us a tour. He showed us around the small campus, and we discussed classes. The veterinary school was tiny, he explained, and there were only seven to twelve students per year. I was impressed with the facilities, especially for cows, which were one of the main species they worked with. When I asked about the potential for a student exchange program, Langa was hesitant.

The students would need to vote, he explained. The issue was that Nelson Mandela had called for an international boycott of South Africa to exert pressure on the government to end apartheid. An exchange program would go against the boycott, and he doubted any student would vote against Mandela's request. I was struck by their dedication to Mandela's plan.

Ultimately, the students did vote against a student exchange program. I had failed in my mission to facilitate the program, yet I was glad to understand the reason and to know that although the students could not yet vote in national elections due to their race, they could vote among themselves to make important decisions. I had enormous respect for Langa and his fellow students.

I had a lot to think about during the long flights back to Boston. This time I traveled alone, as my father needed to stay in Johannesburg a bit longer for work. I wondered when I would see my South African family again and hoped it would not be as long as another seven years. I didn't know then that I'd be returning sooner than I could have imagined.

As the plane touched down in Rabat, Morocco, a few months later, I wondered what I had signed up for: spending the summer with someone I'd never met, in a tiny town in northern Africa that I'd never heard of before this trip. My two large suitcases in the hold contained a sleeping bag, modest clothing to cover my shoulders and knees in the desert heat, and several pounds of M&M's.

Fortunately, Carolyn, the vet I'd be living and working with for two months, was warm and welcoming. She was also a powerhouse of energy and had spent the past year organizing a program to test local cattle for the zoonotic disease tuberculosis, in addition to treating all the animals in the small town where she lived. Carolyn had a passion for international development work, which in veterinary terms involves helping people in developing countries by helping their animals (typically food animals). It was something I wanted to explore during my visit, as I found myself drawn to the interconnected relationships between animals and people, and how animals were an integral part of our world.

After a few days, Carolyn and I left Rabat, and after an overnight train ride followed by a four-hour bus ride, we disembarked in the tiny town of Tendrara. It was such a small place that even people in Rabat hadn't heard of it ("Tangier?" "No, *Tendrara*."). As the bus trundled away, I realized that nothing looked familiar, not the style of buildings, the landscape, nor the people's clothing. Carolyn arranged for a donkey cart to carry my suitcases as I tried to adjust to the sensation of being stared at like an item in a shopwindow. I felt overwhelmed, isolated by my differences. I clearly did not belong.

Every day I followed Carolyn around as she tended the town's animals. This was a time-consuming process, as each visit involved a long social component including several cups of mint tea. Women who were veiled and covered when I saw them outside wore colorful clothing in their homes and welcomed us warmly. Most people communicated in Arabic, which Carolyn spoke fairly well, although I was sometimes able to communicate in my rudimentary French. I did learn a few words of Arabic, common terms for things like *okay, thanks, thank you very much, hot*, and *dust storm*. I learned to live with having electricity and running water for only a part of the day. It was comforting, how I needed less than I'd thought.

One day, Carolyn and I were called to visit a sheep belonging to a man who lived in the town. The sheep had a tumor, and even as a student, I could tell the prognosis was poor. Carolyn communicated this to the ram's owner, who was visibly upset. Although the conversation was in Arabic and I couldn't tell what they were saying, I could tell from his body language that the owner was distraught, and not simply due to the loss of income that would result from the death of his sheep. Even though his animal was never meant to be a pet, the owner was genuinely attached to him. The herders I met in Morocco were mostly proud, strong men, intimidating at first glance. This man was no different, which is why it came as such a surprise to see him on the verge of tears over the loss of what was essentially a farm animal.

It was the first time I had ever been present when bad news was delivered to someone about their animal. It was hard to watch the herder try to absorb the news. He didn't seem to want to believe it and kept asking Carolyn questions. Later, Carolyn explained to me that she told the man that even if he were in the nearest city, Oujda, or in the capital, Rabat, or even in America, there would be no medicine to fix his sheep. There was nothing to do now but to grieve the loss.

My research project involved interviewing the nomadic herders that lived outside the town. We used my grant money to hire a Land Rover and an Arabic-to-French interpreter so that we could meet people who were located far from one another and better understand the nuances of our Arabic conversations. Interviews took place in the herders' tents, where we were treated like guests of honor as we discussed the diseases of their sheep and goats. The herders, living in tandem with their animals, were very knowledgeable about the animals in their care. Carolyn and I were impressed with their understanding of anatomy and their descriptions of the illnesses that befell their animals. This left a deep impression on me, especially the way the stories of human and animal were intertwined, and how their survival depended upon each other.

Near the end of my trip, we were invited to the wedding of a nomadic herder. When we arrived, Carolyn was whisked off by a group of men to examine and admire a prized horse. I tagged along and watched for a while, but Carolyn didn't have time to translate conversations from Arabic to English, so I grew bored. I could hear singing nearby, and I followed the noise to discover a large tent filled with dancing women dressed in brightly colored traditional clothing. An old woman, her face gloriously wrinkled, saw me standing outside and invited me in. She pinched my sundress and examined it, wrinkling her nose at my clearly unsuitable attire, then shook her head and welcomed me anyway.

When Carolyn eventually came looking for me, she was amazed to find me in the middle of the tent, smiling and laughing, surrounded by women, all of us dancing, dancing together. The experience was a highlight of my trip and reminded me that as much as I could consume myself with the needs of animals, and could make their lives my passion, the people in their lives mattered, too.

3

Sacrifices

I returned from Morocco to begin classes at the veterinary campus. Daiquiri and I moved from our fourth-floor city apartment to a house shared with other veterinary students near the school. The house's large yard and access to nearby wooded trails had been a major selling point of the new place. I was finally able to get a dog.

Her name was Trudy. She was a black-and-brindle shelter puppy, and she was bursting with energy and sweet licks on the face that constantly made me smile. With her and Daiquiri, my family felt complete. Every day, Trudy and I walked in the nearby woods together. Whereas before I might have seen a hike as a time to think through an academic problem that had been plaguing me, when walking with Trudy, I saw the world through her senses, watching as she reacted to a cracking branch or a smell hidden from my nose.

I soon found that Trudy was a highly intelligent dog, and she responded well to the hand signals my friend Karen had taught me to use for *sit* and *stay*—she had gotten a golden retriever named

Benjamin a year earlier and knew much more about dog training than I did. If I spotted a turtle in the pond by the trail, Trudy was able to sit noiselessly while I watched for a moment. She trotted by my heels, never straying far off the trail. Trudy loved to retrieve, and much of my limited leisure time was given over to throwing sticks or tennis balls for her. As she grew, one of her large German shepherd–style ears stood up, while the other flopped over. It gave her a distinctly lopsided appearance, and my father liked to joke that she was a rare left-eared African shepherd (the right-eared variety being far more common).

Part of our third-year curriculum involved a "live" or "terminal" surgery lab. Our teachers told us that a crucial part of developing competent surgical techniques was to learn the feel of working with "live tissue" as opposed to practicing on cadavers. One dog per student was used in the labs, and they were humanely euthanized after the procedures. My veterinary school was ahead of the curve as they did make another option available to students, which was rare at the time. Students could opt out of the surgery lab if we agreed to meet certain conditions. However, the alternative program was new and controversial, and the requirements stringent. Only a handful of my classmates opted for the exemption.

I struggled with my decision. It did not seem right to me that a dog had to die for me to become a veterinarian. I did not want to be the cause of a dog's death. But most of our teachers were opposed to the exemption and encouraged us to do the surgeries. Ultimately, I decided to participate in the regular program.

Massachusetts bans pound seizure laws. Dogs impounded as strays were not allowed to be used for experiments or in programs such as the veterinary surgery labs, even if those dogs were not claimed or adopted and were slated for euthanasia anyway. The law was enacted to prevent pets from being treated as lab animals. Our dogs were thus "purpose-bred," which means they were born and bred in lab facilities specifically to be purchased for use in labs and other programs.

Our dogs—beagles—arrived at the school a week or so before the labs, and my classmates and I were required to perform daily physical exams on them. When we went to meet them, our dogs huddled in the backs of their cages. They did not try to bite but seemed unused to human contact. Although they looked like regular dogs, they did not act like them, which deeply saddened me and my friends in the class. My dog did not wag her tail, nor look at me, though I tried to befriend her. She seemed to know that ours would be an awkward relationship. I tried to convey my emotions in my touch as I patted her and in my voice as I spoke to her.

It felt strange to see my surgery dog and then go home to my own dog. Why was one dog's life worth more than another's? The thought plagued me.

I wasn't the only one. My classmates, who before had been eagerly soaking up our lessons and asking thoughtful questions about our readings, would come to class looking sallow and forlorn. More than once I talked with a classmate about how barbaric this was. It felt like some kind of arcane initiation ritual that should have been outlawed long ago. And yet, if we wanted to be vets, we had to go through with it.

Back then, no one spoke to veterinary students about how to cope with thoughts and emotions raised by our surgery labs or by euthanasia in general. The field of veterinary social work had not yet been invented, and there were no counselors or other resources on campus. Our ethics class the year before had not covered this topic and the questions it raised.

The message seemed clear: we needed to be able to handle traumatic and ethically complex situations on our own, without support. Learning to be stoic in the face of emotional stress was simply a part of the curriculum, like taking exams or being sleep-deprived on clinics the day after an overnight hospital shift. If we couldn't handle veterinary school, the message seemed to be, how could we handle veterinary practice?

At the time, I didn't think about being stoic. My classmates and I had all made sacrifices to achieve our dreams of being veterinarians. This was another hoop to jump through, a particularly painful one, which left a scar I wouldn't touch for many years.

The only levity during that difficult time came from an unexpected source: Trudy. The night before one of our lab days, I went to bed early but was awakened by strange beeping noises in my room. I then heard a voice in my room—it was saying, "Hello? Hello?" I realized what must have happened: I shared a desk-style phone with my roommate across the hallway, which we dragged back and forth on a long cord. It was currently on the floor of my room. Trudy had accidentally stepped on the phone—and dialed a number. I got out of bed and quickly hung up. I glanced at the clock; it was 2:00 a.m.

The next morning, I told my three roommates what had happened. Bart, who owned the phone, was busy thinking of his preprogrammed list of family members. I thought I had last spoken to my father, but I knew it wasn't his voice I'd heard. It was a mystery. But we had to focus on the lab day, so we headed to school.

That day, one of my lab partners was doing surgery, and my job was to monitor anesthesia. It was tedious work; we were relieved when lunchtime arrived and we were able to take a break. As I gathered my books to head to the on-campus cafeteria, I overheard a conversation between two of my friends.

"Why are you so tired?" Craig asked Arnaldo after he gave a giant yawn.

"It's weird, but my phone rang last night at two in the morning, and I couldn't get back to sleep."

I doubled over with laughter and turned to face my classmates, who looked at me curiously.

"Did *you* call me?" asked Arnaldo.

"No," I answered, barely getting the words out, "but I know who did!"

Bart had called Arnaldo the night before, and Trudy must have pressed redial, we concluded. Fortunately, Arnaldo was a good friend with an excellent sense of humor and readily accepted my apology. We laughed even harder when Arnaldo reminded us that his girlfriend Naiomi was visiting from Puerto Rico; what had she thought of the early-morning call? "I'll have to tell her," Arnaldo joked, "that it was just some dog who called me." My friend was not the type to be disrespectful to women, and we imagined Naiomi's surprise as the caller's identity was revealed.

When it was my turn for the surgery lab, I tried to get as much out of the experience as I could. I wanted my dog's death to help me as much as possible, so I could help other animals. The dog was under anesthesia for several hours as my lab partners and I performed several different procedures on her, learning the feel of internal organs and tissues, practicing surgical techniques so we wouldn't be performing them for the first time on someone's pet. At the end of the day, while still under anesthesia, she would be euthanized right there on the table, through her intravenous catheter.

When the time came, I was ready to accept my responsibility. The veterinary technician who had assisted our lab group produced a labeled syringe full of bright pink euthanasia solution. The dog lay on her side on the table, mostly covered by surgical drapes. I reached underneath and patted her for the last time, mentally apologizing for what I was about to do. Then, I faced the technician.

"I can do it," I said, reaching for the syringe, accepting my fate as well as the dog's.

"No," said the technician. I was surprised, but she was firm. "I'll do it."

It was a simple matter of inserting the needle through the rubber stopper of the catheter and depressing the plunger. Yet the result was the death of "my" dog. Had the technician been instructed to administer the euthanasia solution, or had she taken it upon herself to prevent me from doing it? I never found out. But I am grateful to her for sparing me a portion of suffering on that difficult day. Although the dog died because of me, I didn't have to euthanize her myself.

Fortunately, there has been progress. Tufts eliminated terminal surgery labs a few years after I graduated, the first veterinary school in the United States to do so. Terminal surgeries have been phased out at many veterinary schools, and they instead partner with animal shelters to allow veterinary students, supervised by clinicians, to spay and neuter adoptable pets, creating a win-win situation: the students gain surgical experience on live tissue, and shelter pets get neutered. Many veterinary students no longer need to agonize over whether a dog must lose a life for them to graduate.

One day, my father called with bad news: Oupa had been diagnosed with Lou Gehrig's disease, or ALS—rare at his age of seventy-nine. It was a devastating diagnosis, and as a physician, he knew just how the disease would progress. He would slowly lose mobility, and the condition was ultimately fatal. My father arranged for me to travel to South Africa during my spring break. I knew it would be my last visit with my grandfather.

Oupa was still seeing the occasional patient in a room in my grandparents' apartment, despite needing to use a scooter. He'd have the patient get on his bed, and he would listen with his stethoscope and take their pulse. He gently examined the eczema on my hands just as he always did when I saw him. He couldn't help himself; being a doctor was a part of his identity. I'd brought Oupa a medical book about ALS, and he read through it carefully. I was still in school, but he made me feel like a colleague, a fellow "medical person" who understood how he craved information about his condition. I knew I would miss this mutual understanding and collegiality when he was gone.

One day, a patient of his came by with a gift: a bottle of Oupa's favorite Scotch whiskey.

"Hooch!" said my grandfather, brightening visibly. His patients knew him well. Oupa loved to have one small glass per day of whiskey and water.

This visit felt different, and a sadness permeated the air. I couldn't interest Granny in her favorite card game, gin rummy. Oupa was upset because he was struggling to eat with utensils. It was becoming difficult for him to hold them, and he kept dropping his food, often staining his shirt. I tried to cheer him up.

"Hilary told me that yesterday she spilled coffee on herself at work and it was so bad that she had to go home and change," I told him. We laughed together, but we knew why he was struggling and that it would only get worse.

I nibbled a piece of dark chocolate from the plate Granny had placed on the table. My family's natural end to a meal was a Cadbury bar broken into squares.

"Tell the story," I begged my grandmother, "about how you went to Nairobi to see Oupa." It was my favorite story, and Granny loved to tell it. During World War II, Oupa had enlisted as a medic and was based in Nairobi, although he was sometimes sent farther north.

Granny settled in to tell her tale. "I went to the army headquarters in Johannesburg with Hazel, who was three at the time, and I told them I wouldn't leave until they put me on a troop transport to Nairobi so I could see my husband."

My grandmother was known in our family not for her cooking

nor her charm but for her persistence. The army had indeed allowed them onto a plane, and it had taken a few days to travel to Nairobi, as the airplane was allowed to fly only at night for safety.

"We arrived in Nairobi, but your grandfather wasn't there. We weren't allowed to contact him, but you see, there was a man who worked at the post office who was from Johannesburg, and he knew Morrie. So he got word to your oupa that his wife and daughter were waiting for him in Nairobi. And I waited and waited," said my grandmother. "Hazel and I stayed at a hotel. Every day, a man came around to bring tea. And one day there was a knock on the door, and I said, 'You can come in with the tea,' and it was your oupa!" Granny's eyes twinkled as they always did at the memory, as did Oupa's.

Something struck me then that had never occurred to me before, despite all the times I'd heard the story.

"Granny, Hazel was three," I said, thinking out loud, "and she's four years older than my father . . ."

"That's right!" Granny laughed. "Your father was conceived there!"

My family was even more international than I had thought.

After the trip, I felt disoriented; I'd been gone for only ten days but it seemed like much longer. Some classmates had traveled for spring break, while others had stayed home. No one else, it seemed, had journeyed to the other side of the world to visit a beloved family member for the last time. I kept thinking about life, and death, and how I would miss my grandfather's voice. I felt different in a fundamental way, while nothing around me had changed.

Soon, it was time to begin "clinics"; our classroom work was finished, and our class was moving on to clinical rotations. There was no summer break between third and fourth years. There was a lottery for rotation schedules, with results eagerly anticipated. I had chosen to put the large animal ambulatory rotation into the lottery. It was a monthlong rotation with the Tufts Ambulatory Service, a group of veterinarians in Connecticut, about forty-five minutes away, who treated mainly cows and the occasional sheep or goat. I knew we'd be spending most of the time outdoors or in unheated barns, and I wanted to do the rotation in the warmer months, as I dreaded doing it in winter. I was glad to have gotten my choice.

There were four veterinarians who ran the program, all men. One was known for his friendly demeanor and for stopping at McDonald's with his students, treating them to a cup of coffee and relaxed conversation. The others were more businesslike.

It felt good to be back on a dairy farm again. The atmosphere was comforting and familiar; the scent of raw milk, the scraping of my knee-high boots on the concrete floor of the milk room, the shiny-clean stainless steel of the milk storage tanks, the low moos of the cows, the swishing tails and the smell of manure.

One of the things we needed to learn on the rotation was how to check cows for pregnancy, a basic skill for a farm-animal vet. This involved a rectal examination. We were shown how to put on an arm-length clear plastic sleeve and fasten it to the shoulder of our coveralls. After generously applying lubricant, we'd stand behind a cow and begin by slowly and carefully removing any manure, using our hand as a scoop, and letting it drop to the manure trough below. Finally, we were ready to feel for the cow's reproductive organs through the wall of the rectum and check for pregnancy.

It was a change from putting milking machines on the cows, which they were used to from being milked twice daily. I was now standing directly behind them, making myself vulnerable to a kick from one of their large hooves. And while I generally didn't mind the smell of cow manure, I was awfully close to an awful lot of it. Otherwise, I was game to learn a new skill. So much of our education had been based on things we needed to memorize and understand with our minds; it was refreshing to be trained in something physical.

My problem was height. At just under five foot two, I was the shortest one on the rotation. I could scoop out the manure, but inserting my arm involved reaching upward. Palpating for pregnancy involved feeling downward on the floor of the rectum. Reaching up and then down was challenging and effectively shortened my arm length so that I was unable to feel what we were supposed to locate. When I asked the professors for suggestions, they just shrugged. I longed to ask for some sort of accommodation like a stool to stand on, but I didn't want to be labeled as "that student." So I did the best I could, and when a tall male student commented excitedly near the end of the rotation that he was really getting the hang of the pregnancy checks, I was jealous but held my tongue.

One day, we stopped at a barn to check on a sick cow and the farmer asked about a newborn calf that hadn't been eating well.

"Oh, well, that's a job for your wife," responded the veterinarian with a grin, indicating that the male farmer didn't need to bother himself with something so unimportant. "You know, women have those nurturing hormones. Just tell her to bottle-feed it."

Back in the truck, I couldn't help myself. "So what exactly are those 'nurturing hormones' that women have?" I asked. I wasn't surprised when he laughed it off, but it was important to me that he knew I considered it a sexist remark. How could women expect to be taken seriously as doctors if they were pigeonholed into gender roles and "women's work" was denigrated? And what about men's ability or desire to nurture?

During my fourth year, I also traveled to the Navajo Nation in Arizona. There was a clinic on the reservation with an elective program that hosted senior veterinary students from different schools. We bunked in a few rooms with mattresses in a loft above the large-animal section of the hospital. This was convenient because we didn't need a car; however, it also meant that students worked long hours as we were always available to see patients and perform treatments.

On the bus from the airport in Albuquerque, I was glued to the window. I had never visited the southwestern United States before and was struck by the wide vistas, so different from the shady hills and valleys of New England. After a couple of hours, I got off at the bus stop closest to the clinic, where I was met by another veterinary student. She was from the Pacific Northwest and had been sent to pick me up as she had her own car.

At the clinic, I met a newly graduated veterinarian who had a wonderful little dog named Katrina that went everywhere with him. Every so often she limped on one of her back legs, and although she seemed hardly bothered by the limp, I noticed her owner wince each time, as if he were the one in pain.

One day, I asked him about it. He told me that the state where he attended veterinary school had not banned its pound seizure law. His veterinary class had performed surgeries on shelter dogs slated for euthanasia. Katrina had been his surgery dog, and he had performed an unnecessary surgery on her back leg. Rather than euthanize her afterward, he'd adopted her, which was forbidden at my school. Although his surgery dog had lived, they both bore scars from the experience.

One of the patients under my care at the Navajo clinic was Snowball, a snow-white kitty who had been brought into the clinic with a broken leg. An X-ray revealed that the leg was badly fractured and would be impossible to repair. The best option was amputation.

Amputation. It's a loaded word. People tend to think of amputation as a pretty big deal. How would this little cat react, I wondered?

It was 1991, and the clinic did not have the latest anesthesia products, so Snowball was under anesthesia for a long time. She did well through the surgery but slept a lot the following day. By the next day, the now three-legged cat was more awake. She purred in her cage, appearing more comfortable than she had been before the surgery, when her leg had been causing her only pain.

That day, I picked Snowball up and brought her out of her cage. After examining her incision to make sure it was healing well, I gently placed her onto the floor to see what she would do. Snowball seemed to take it in stride that she now had only three legs. She wobbled occasionally as she adjusted to her new physical condition and tried to balance. And then off she went. It was day three, and the little cat was walking, eating, and purring. I wondered how many people would do so well just a few days after an amputation.

Snowball's rapid adjustment made me appreciate how much of our stress can be mental. Any person post-amputation might well be thinking about all the things they will miss, how hard their life is about to become, and how others will view them, among other things. Snowball was distracted by none of those thoughts. She accepted her condition as it was *in that moment* and adjusted accordingly.

I also considered the term *mentally prepared*. Had Snowball prepared mentally for her amputation? Not likely. However, I developed a theory. Snowball was aware her body had sustained a serious injury; she knew her leg was painful, and she was unable to use it. Perhaps, having completely internalized and accepted that information, she was more able to adapt to the loss of her leg.

It was the first time I started to wonder about the mind-body connection when it came to healing and how, in many cases, it allows a faster recovery. It was my first inkling that we may be able to learn something from how animals react to medical problems. Little did I know how useful such a lesson would be when I experienced my own medical difficulties.

One evening about a month after I returned from the elective in Arizona, my phone rang. It was my father; Oupa was struggling to breathe. I immediately left for my parents' house. When I arrived, my father told me that Granny had called to say the doctor had arrived and wanted to give Oupa morphine to relieve his discomfort, but that he might not survive. She asked my father what to do, and he told her to go ahead. They both knew my grandfather had arranged beforehand for his doctor friend to stop his suffering once Oupa could no longer breathe on his own. My grandfather had not wanted to live out his final days on a ventilator in the hospital, unable to communicate, which was the only other option at the time. He wanted to die at home. We later learned that he had seen a patient the day he died. His mind was 100 percent.

It was something Oupa had done himself for a select few patients. Although Oupa never discussed this with me, he had discussed it with my father, telling him that it was a part of his Hippocratic oath to relieve suffering. He always had long conversations with the patients and arranged a signal for when the patient felt it was time. Although euthanasia was illegal in South Africa, my grandfather did it anyway. I imagined a terminally ill patient touching my grandfather's hand and asking for a peaceful death when the time came, and Oupa agreeing. It was a fact that would help me make sense of my own conflicted feelings about euthanasia and to make peace with them. I knew that the ability to provide a peaceful death and end suffering was a blessing.

My father began packing for an early-morning flight. He had arranged to meet up with his sister from Chicago, my aunt Hazel, in New York, so they could travel to Johannesburg together.

Back in my apartment the next day, it felt strange to be so far away, unable to gather with family after my grandfather's death. I wasn't going to take a day off, but after I spoke to Karen, I decided to take the day for myself. I was on an elective, and my teacher was understanding. I grieved with my immediate family, Trudy and Daiquiri, bringing Trudy on a long, quiet walk.

As my father and aunt sorted through Oupa's possessions in South Africa, they decided that I should inherit his doctor bag, the one he used for house calls. Even now, all these years later, it is one of my most prized possessions: a vintage brown briefcase with brass fasteners and an outside pocket for folders and papers. The bag opened into two covered halves, each containing multiple compartments. Inside were some of Oupa's medical instruments: a small forceps, a hemostat clamp—items he probably used to place sutures but that had many other uses as well. It was a treasure, and I was honored to have it. At the time, I didn't realize it would be a gateway to how I would practice medicine.

As the weather grew colder, I had more rotations inside the hospital. Unfortunately, my allergies emerged again, this time when I was in the large-animal hospital. Every time I went into a horse stall, I sneezed uncontrollably. Someone suggested wearing a dust mask, and it worked. As I walked around the hospital, I was met first with confused expressions and then understanding nods and remarks of "Allergies, huh?"

Most of the large-animal hospital patients were horses, with the occasional sheep or goat. Cows were simply not worth enough money to justify trailering them to the hospital and paying for specialty care. One of the large-animal clinicians was shorter than me, and one day I saw her nonchalantly standing on a stool while examining a horse. It made me wish I had spoken up during my ambulatory rotation.

During the small-animal surgery rotation, I met a frail elderly woman, Mrs. Anderson, with a mastiff named Athena. Mastiffs are enormous dogs, and Athena easily outweighed me as well as her owner. At first glance, Athena and Mrs. Anderson seemed an odd pair. However, I was about to learn how closely they were bonded to each other.

Athena was friendly and let me take her temperature, pulse, and respiration. I interviewed her owner about the reason for the appointment before going to find the clinician. Athena, it turned out, needed surgery on her knee ligament and had been referred to Tufts by her regular veterinarian. Although most dogs were able to return home within a couple of days of the surgery, Mrs. Anderson was worried about taking Athena outdoors during the recovery period. Athena had stairs to navigate at home, and snow was forecasted for the following week. It was safer, she felt, to have Athena stay at the hospital for a couple of weeks until she was more mobile. After everything was settled with the surgeon, I led Athena off to set up a nice large run in the dog ward of the hospital. I was relieved to discover that she walked easily on leash and didn't try to drag me off down the hospital corridor.

Athena was my case, so each morning I was required to arrive early at the hospital to examine her and write my findings in her medical chart. She did well through the surgery, and I grew fond of the giant dog and looked forward to seeing her each morning. About halfway through Athena's stay, I finished my surgery rotation. I gave Athena a pat, telling her that my next rotation was also in the small-animal hospital so I would come and visit her. She would become another student's case for the remainder of her stay.

A couple of days later, I visited Athena in the dog ward. I was shocked to discover large signs taped across the chain-link door to her run: CAUTION—WILL BITE—DO NOT ENTER. I found one of the technicians and asked her about it.

"*That* dog? She tried to take a student's face off!" she responded. "They can barely get near her."

"Athena?" I was incredulous. "She's always been fine with me." I opened Athena's door, cautious after hearing the news about my friend. Athena wagged her tail and allowed me to pat her giant head. Nothing had changed between us.

From then on, I tried to find time in the morning to help Athena's new student with her daily exam. One afternoon, I was paged to go to the treatment area in the ward. I found Athena lying down, surrounded by the surgery resident and several students. The resident was trying to remove Athena's sutures, but the dog refused to let anyone near her leg. I spoke to Athena in soothing tones as I patted her and slowly approached. She lay calmly and allowed me to touch her leg. The resident handed me the suture scissors and I easily removed the dog's sutures as I had been taught, making sure not to leave part of the suture material inside.

As gratifying as it was to be called off my current rotation to work on a patient only I could handle, I suspected Athena's preference wasn't really about me personally. What was special about me, I wondered, that would allow the dog to trust me and no one else? Everyone there loved animals. No one had been unkind or rough with Athena. The only difference about me, I realized, was that I had met Athena with her owner present. Mrs. Anderson had permitted me to examine Athena and lead her out of the room. She had essentially given me her blessing, allowing her loyal dog to trust me.

Fortunately, after the suture removal, Athena was deemed mobile enough to return home to Mrs. Anderson. I imagined their happy reunion. Although they had initially appeared to be a mismatched pair, I sensed the love—and trust—between them. They were family.

————

As the end of fourth year approached, it was time to look for a job. I had been so struck by the landscape of the Southwest that I decided to return to New Mexico to try to find a job there. The Navajo Nation elective had mentioned a stipend of $400 if the participant submitted an essay after their experience. I submitted my essay and the money was enough for a plane ticket to Albuquerque for me and Trudy (as it was cheaper for me to bring her than to board her). Trudy and I stayed in youth hostels and a motel when no single room was available in the hostel.

There was one job possibility I was excited about. It involved driving an RV into a Native American reservation two days a week and staying overnight, treating a population that lived far from existing veterinary clinics. I imagined myself taking the RV into the wilderness, Trudy at my side, treating animals that relied on me for help. In this daydream, I was also taller.

At the job interview, the reality appeared far different from what I had anticipated. I asked about declawing cats, a procedure I did not want to perform. Declawing involves amputating a cat's knuckles, a painful procedure that is never in the cat's best interest. While most clinics performed declaws routinely, many tried to discourage it, educating clients about trimming their kitten's nails and making scratching posts available. The office manager instead informed me that the practice actively encouraged declawing their feline patients; there appeared to be little flexibility in their policy. And although I was prepared to work hard, the RV portion of the job, which I had romanticized, appeared overwhelming when I thought about it more realistically. Each day would involve several hours of driving in addition to a full day of seeing patients. There would be no support staff and no opportunity for communication with the clinic. The job did not seem like a good fit for a brand-new graduate, and I wondered whether they were trying to take advantage of the naivete of young veterinarians.

After the interview, I spoke to my parents, disappointed that the opportunity I had been excited about seemed problematic up close.

"All jobs will have their issues," my mother advised. "You find out about them after you start working there. If a job seems to have difficulties before you even start, that's not a good sign." I knew she was right.

I had sent resumes to other clinics who had advertised for a veterinarian, and I followed up with phone calls. At one clinic, the owner answered the phone himself. When I told him who I was and asked if he had received my resume, he laughed.

"Oh, I won't hire a woman," he told me firmly.

The words seemed to echo inside my head. "Excuse me?" I asked. I couldn't possibly have heard correctly.

"I'm not going to bother training a woman who's just going to get pregnant and quit."

After all the years of hard work and sacrifice, the words were devastating. I was being denied an opportunity simply due to my gender. Although I tried to comfort myself by thinking that I wouldn't want to work for such a jerk anyway, it was sobering to realize that certain jobs in my field were simply inaccessible. Despite the large number of women in my class, most veterinary practice owners were men. How many of them, I wondered, shared that veterinarian's feelings about hiring women? Small business owners could do as they liked. For some jobs, apparently, I wasn't just at a disadvantage; I wasn't even in the running.

Fortunately, not all my future colleagues were so unpleasant. One veterinarian, a Dr. Riegger, took the time to send me a handwritten notecard saying that he wasn't currently hiring but would keep my resume on file and I was welcome to stop by for a visit. The card had a white-and-yellow flower on the front, a painting by Georgia O'Keeffe, and I pulled it out often to remind myself that kindness existed.

When I returned to Massachusetts, the annual convention of the American Veterinary Medical Association (AVMA) was being held in Boston. It was a rare opportunity to attend a large national conference without having to travel, and I was excited to go. At the convention center, I attended lectures and browsed exhibit halls, still in disbelief that I was a full-fledged doctor. The convention held the most veterinarians I had ever seen in one place, and the demographics were startling. About half the doctors near my age were women. Yet veterinarians who looked to be forty or older were almost exclusively male. I didn't know it then, but the convention also included a seventy-fifth-anniversary celebration of the Auxiliary to the AVMA. The group, called the Women's Auxiliary until 1977, was formed by wives to support their veterinarian husbands. Until recently, the closest most women could get to veterinary medicine was to marry a doctor. Now I was on the edge of a new wave of female practitioners. Despite the discrimination I'd already faced on my job search, I felt fortunate to be a part of the profession, and grateful to the brave women who had gone before me.

4

Ain't Doin' Right

Since I couldn't find a job in New Mexico, I found one back in Massachusetts, and after graduation began working in a small-animal practice. This had been my dream for so long and I was thrilled to finally have the chance to do it. I was excited to use my medical knowledge and I loved seeing animals all day, but I was surprised by how much I appreciated listening to people's stories about their pets and witnessing firsthand how much they loved their animals. While I hadn't wanted to work with people about their own medical problems, I found tremendous enjoyment talking with people about their pets. Working at a small-animal practice also introduced me to many of the challenges and joys of working with animals full-time.

My first job out of vet school was at an animal clinic, where, each week, I worked four ten-hour shifts and was on call two nights for emergencies. It was very much being thrown in the deep end, where sinking meant potentially doing harm to an animal under my care. I had no choice but to swim.

My days at the clinic were spent mostly seeing patients. Every fifteen minutes I would have another appointment. I would see that a new patient had come into the office by the colored folder placed on the rack in the wall. When a new folder arrived, I would read through it, glancing at the history the person at reception had taken. Then I would go into the waiting room to call the patient and client into an exam room.

During these days, I saw mostly cats and dogs. They had lumps on their torsos or digestive problems. They were losing weight or gaining weight, had personality changes or were just there for wellness checks. Every time I doubted my diagnosis, I would make an excuse about needing to take the animal to the treatment room out back, "where the light is better." Then I would consult with one of the other three doctors who worked there, all women, to make sure I made the right call.

Meanwhile, I was constantly talking. To the patients. To the owners. To the staff members who were helping me. Even during my lunch break, which everyone took together in the break room, I was talking. I would call owners who had phoned during the day with questions. I would call clients to talk through test results that had come back. I would call to check in on patients I had already seen. The one time, however, I knew not to talk was from one to two every day. That was sacred time, reserved for *All My Children.*

The three other veterinarians (along with the receptionists and technicians) were adamant that I not ruin a single second of *All My Children* with my chatter. Even if I didn't understand the appeal of the show, I knew better than to break this cardinal rule. Finally, I began asking questions about characters and plotlines during the commercials: Was that guy's name Ted or Tad? How many ex-husbands does Erica have anyway? Does the same actor really play Adam and Stuart? At least then I could begin to understand some of the show's improbable story lines.

One day a week, however, I didn't see any patients. This was a day reserved for surgeries. Most of the time the surgery would be a spay, a neuter, or removing a lump. While today, vets have more oversight and assistance, back then I was by myself in a surgery room doing practically everything.

I would start by injecting the patient with an anesthetic, while an assistant helped hold the animal. Then I would insert an endotracheal tube into the animal's airway and attach it to the anesthesia machine, which administered inhalant anesthetics. The assistant or a technician would then shave the fur around the surgical area and apply an antiseptic while I scrubbed in for the procedure, washing my hands with the special sponge brush and antiseptic solution used by both human and veterinary surgeons to make myself as germ-free as possible before putting on sterile gloves.

Today most veterinarians have a certified technician remain in the room with them to monitor anesthesia and assist the surgeon by handing them suture material from a sterile package when required. Back then, I had to yell out if I needed something. When I heard the techs whispering and smiling one day, I insisted they reveal the joke. "You don't yell loud enough," they told me, "so we've been saying that only dogs can hear you." I found this hysterical, but I did try to yell louder when I needed help after that.

The hardest part of my job, though, was not the surgeries. It was the nights I was on call for emergencies. I would get a call in the middle of the night through the answering service. I would return the call and talk with distraught owners about whatever problems their animals had that the owners were concerned enough about to feel the need for immediate care.

I would meet these owners and animals at the clinic in the middle of the night. I was by myself. I had no one to consult. I was constantly afraid of making the wrong call. What I remember most about those early days was the constant fear. Everything felt like life and death then. In many ways, it was.

Often, I sensed uncertainty from clients about my capabilities, likely based on a combination of my gender and my youth. I was twenty-five when I graduated and began working but apparently looked younger. When I went to get my hair cut at a local salon, the stylist asked me conversationally, "So, do you go to the high school?" I blamed it on the jean overalls I was wearing but never went back.

A few months into my first job, a woman came in with her young daughter and their cat.

"Look, Jessica, a lady doctor, a doctor for animals!" said the mother as she entered the exam room. I swelled with pride.

Jessica eyed me skeptically. "Girls can't be doctors," she informed us.

Mom appeared as shocked as I was, and we fell over ourselves to convince Jessica that girls certainly *can* be doctors.

When I sensed doubt from a client, I worked hard to win them over. Usually, by the time an appointment ended, I earned a grudging attitude I interpreted as *she seems to know what she's talking about.*

Clients weren't the only ones I had to convince of my competence. I also had to convince my coworkers. The receptionists, assistants, technicians, and doctors knew I had just graduated. But it soon came to light that there was one important thing I had not learned in veterinary school. A basic thing: how to express anal glands.

Anal glands, also called anal sacs, are small glands just inside the anus of dogs and cats. They fill with a noxious-smelling material, and in some dogs (and, more rarely, some cats) they can become full and uncomfortable, so they need to be squeezed, or expressed. This requires a glove, some lubricant, and at least one person to hold the dog, as the procedure is unpleasant and most dogs squirm or even try to bite. Anal gland material is extremely stinky, although not as bad as those animals famous for their anal gland scent: skunks.

Expressing anal glands is certainly not the most glamorous part of veterinary work, but it is called for often. You could say it's one of the bread-and-butter tasks, like nail trims.

In veterinary school, I had learned how to place an intravenous catheter, identify different types of cells and parasites under a microscope, and utilize different kinds of suturing techniques. It was probably assumed that I would learn such basic skills as anal gland expression at the clinics I worked at on my elective weeks. Yet most clinics would not allow a veterinary student to perform procedures on a client's pet. And so, at least in my case, anal gland expression had fallen through the cracks.

My veterinary colleagues, who had also been to veterinary school, likely didn't judge me for needing to learn this fundamental skill. The staff was another story. As far as they were concerned, if I had arrived not knowing how to perform the most basic of tasks, one that technicians and many veterinary assistants knew how to do, how likely was I to know more complicated things?

When the receptionist came back to the treatment area one day and stated that a client was on the phone asking whether her dog could have given her children lice, I knew the answer. "No, it's not possible, because lice are species-specific. They don't travel to other species," I explained. But the receptionist looked right past me to the other doctor, waiting to hear her confirmation before talking to the client.

I had to work to be taken seriously by my coworkers as well as by my clients, and all too often, I doubted myself. Only my patients fully accepted me.

The first clinic I worked at still handled a few of the shrinking population of local dairy farms. One day, near the end of my shift, I was sent out on a farm call for a cow emergency.

A cow had a prolapsed uterus. Although I had never treated a cow before, I knew that a prolapsed uterus could be an issue for cows after they deliver a calf.

As I drove to the farm, I went over what I remembered from school. The uterus would be swollen, and it would be at least partially outside the cow's body. My job would be to try to push the large organ back inside the cow where it belonged. Sugar could shrink the swelling, and I was to apply that liberally. My teachers had stressed to not even attempt to replace a uterus unless the cow was lying sternal, on its stomach, not on its side. I knew I had my work cut out for me.

At the farm, a teenager showed me the cow. She was lying on her side on a mound of hay in the muddy farmyard. I could tell that she had been down for some time, as the uterus was completely externalized and very swollen. When I saw her, I immediately felt a pang in my chest.

"She's old anyways," the farmer told me when he arrived. I didn't like his casual tone. "But see what you can do." He spun on his heel and left.

The cow didn't seem uncomfortable, but her uterus needed to get back inside her body if she was to survive. The teenager and I, with the help of a small backhoe, did our best to keep the cow sternal, and we liberally applied the sugar I had brought with me from the clinic. The uterus was larger than the cow's head and weighed at least forty pounds. As I tried to push the organ back into the cow's body, I realized, to my horror, that the tissue was friable. That is, it was tearing easily. It was already damaged, despite the care I was taking to be gentle.

I spent hours trying to push the uterus back inside the cow, stopping every now and then to apply sugar. However, even though I was covered in sweat (and other juices), I was getting nowhere. At last I had to acknowledge that it was time to stop.

I drove home, crying all the way. It was my first farm call, and I had failed miserably. The poor cow would be sold for slaughter.

When I got home to Trudy and Daiquiri, I made chocolate chip cookies to cheer myself up. After a couple of cookies, I needed a glass of milk. Standing in front of the open refrigerator, I took one look at the milk container and burst into tears.

Now, as a more-experienced vet, I can look back on that event and see that I never could have saved that cow. The farmer had called me too late. But back then, as green as I was, when I didn't know my own capabilities and was overly afraid of doing damage to the creatures under my care, I was heartbroken.

The cow was an either-or situation: fix the problem or the animal would be euthanized. However, I was learning that for many animals, there were different options for diagnosis and treatment, depending on what an owner could afford. Although veterinary medicine is an excellent value compared with human medicine, costs can be prohibitive when paying out of pocket. I began saying to clients, "In an ideal world, money is no object, but we live in the real world" as I helped them make sense of their choices. As a veterinarian, I needed to be conscious of what a client was willing and able to spend, and act accordingly. Most practitioners thus become skilled at trying to work out a plan B for an animal's treatment, or even a plan C, when plan A cannot fit into an owner's budget. This often means we are without a diagnosis and must rely on intuition and experience to treat our patients.

It may help if more pet owners had pet health insurance, or perhaps if this were covered by employers or as part of a health insurance policy. This makes sense because owning a pet has been proven to make us healthier, so why not cover some of the costs? The benefits to having a pet are numerous and profound; a pet should not have to be a luxury item.

While expenses related to food and routine veterinary care are fairly standard, the cost of managing a sudden illness or injury can be substantial. However, some veterinarians worry that pet insurance will become like human health insurance and require practitioners to spend large amounts of time handling claims forms and, worse, even control which medications and treatments are used. This would drive up veterinary prices for everyone.

Early in my career, I had a sweet Doberman patient named Brody who'd begun to have pain upon opening his mouth. I ran some blood tests, which were normal. I dispensed antibiotics, and the problem went away. A month or so later, though, the problem was back, and this time the dog felt even worse. I could tell it really hurt for the poor guy to open his mouth. I knew there could be an abscess or infection causing the pain, but I was also concerned about cancer. At that point, I recommended taking X-rays of Brody's head, and his owner agreed.

Radiographs of the head are challenging to interpret, for several reasons; there are many tiny bones in a small space, making the X-rays difficult to read (especially in the days before digital radiography, which can enlarge images), and most veterinarians don't take them often, so we are not accustomed to evaluating them. Although anything consisting of bone or metal shows up well on an X-ray, other substances can be difficult to differentiate.

I didn't see any obvious issues on Brody's X-rays, but I was concerned I might be missing something, so I called his owner and recommended sending the X-rays to Tufts for the veterinary radiologists to interpret. I also recommended repeating some of the blood tests to see if anything had changed: whether his white blood cell count, which had been normal, had increased, possibly indicating an infection. Brody's owner asked how much each would cost, and I gave him the prices, which were about the same for each of the things I was recommending.

"Well, Doc, I can afford one but not both. I don't know which one to do. You decide," he said.

I thought hard. The blood work would be good to have, certainly. But we had already run blood work, and it could well be normal again, whereas I might get a diagnosis from having his radiographs read by a bona fide radiologist.

I decided to send the X-rays out. With the digital X-ray machines many veterinary practices currently use, sending X-rays out for interpretation involves a simple email, and results can be obtained within hours if needed. Back then, the physical X-ray film had to be sent in the mail or hand-delivered. I placed Brody on some pain medication while we waited for results.

A week or so later, I had my response. The report from Tufts stated that the dog's temporomandibular joint (TMJ) area appeared clear of infection, but the radiologist had noticed a small area on the mandible, or lower jawbone, which looked like it could be a tumor. Unsatisfied, I called the radiologist for clarification. How certain was he? Pretty certain, it turned out. This was not good news to give Brody's owner. However, I was relieved to have made the right decision regarding which test to run. Now we could at least treat Brody for his actual condition. I prescribed some prednisone to help with pain and inflammation, and Brody was able to eat again.

Sometimes I wonder what it must be like to practice with no regard to cost. I always try to do the best for my patients no matter what their owners can afford. And, as my grandfather did with his patients, I try to maximize the information I get from my physical exam and patient history. A typical neighborhood small-animal veterinarian must act as an internal medicine doctor, a surgeon, an anesthesiologist, a radiologist, an ophthalmologist, a dentist, an emergency room doctor, a cardiologist, a dermatologist, a neurologist, a nutritionist, an orthopedist, an oncologist, a pharmacist, a parasitologist, and an animal behaviorist, among other things. I have heard it said that veterinarians who enter specialty professions are doing so to relieve the "boredom" of general practice. Personally, I can't imagine anything less boring.

Although there were specialists available when I first practiced, it was a rare occurrence for one of my clients to seek their services. When I suggested a specialist, I braced for the typical response:

"You want me to bring Scooter to an animal *eye doctor/dermatologist/oncologist?* Is there really such a thing?"

I always wanted people to at least know there was an option of seeing a specialist if I thought it would benefit their pet. Whether they followed up or not was up to them. These days, a client may decline a referral, but they are far less likely to laugh in my face. Most people have heard of veterinary specialists and may have already brought their pet to one or know someone who has. However, it is simply not an option for everyone.

Although sometimes the cause of a problem is obvious, like a prolapsed uterus, a sick animal is often a puzzle to be solved. Sometimes I can figure it out from the history the owner is giving me, or from watching the animal across the room, or from my physical exam. In some cases we need blood tests and X-rays, perhaps followed by more involved, expensive tests such as ultrasounds. At times, a veterinarian will refer a patient to a specialist for a consultation or for more-involved testing such as an MRI, and occasionally, as with human medicine, even specialists may be unable to diagnose the problem.

When I question people about their animals, I know from experience that certain conditions tend to fit into certain patterns. For instance, animals with urinary tract infections typically don't lose their appetites. If I suspect a bladder infection (commonly known as a UTI), but the animal has also stopped eating, I may start thinking of other things, such as a kidney infection.

I undoubtedly rely on the owner's body language as well as that of my patients—one reason I have always disliked "drop-offs." A drop-off is when the receptionist says, "The owner couldn't stay for an appointment, so she dropped her cat off. Here's the chart, and Fluffy is in a cage out back. She has been vomiting and is ADR." *ADR* is a commonly used term in the veterinary profession, and it is a tribute to British veterinarian and author James Herriot. ADR stands for "ain't doing right"—as in, "Well, Doc, I can't put my finger on it, but Lucky's not himself. He just *ain't doin' right.*"

Despite our scientific training, veterinarians tend to be superstitious, and many will tell you that a dog named Lucky could turn out to be anything but, while a cat named Princess or Buttercup may become ferocious when handled.

To figure out how the animal wasn't "right," I'd ask the client about their pet's normal behavior. The owner would then typically tell a story about what their pet was doing that was different: not greeting the person at the door, not staying up late to watch television, or declining to finish their supper. Even these small behavioral changes could be a sign of a serious problem.

I would then need to examine Fluffy, and call the owner to ask a multitude of questions: When did your kitty last vomit? How long has she been vomiting for—hours, days, weeks? How many times a day has she been vomiting? How long after eating? Is it fur or something else? Could she have gotten into anything? Have you changed her diet lately? Does she have diarrhea, too? Have there been any changes in Fluffy's home environment—moving, construction, new pets or people, schedule changes? Does she go outside, or is she strictly an indoor cat?

I may do a fair amount of reading between the lines. How concerned is the owner? Maybe Fluffy vomited on something precious, which triggered the drop-off. Perhaps a family member has been ill and Fluffy is reacting to the stress. Perhaps there is a new puppy who wants to play with the cat, and she has nowhere to hide. Perhaps Fluffy has lost weight recently. The cat could have a foreign body stuck in her digestive tract, a hyperactive thyroid gland, kidney disease, an allergy, cancer, inflammatory bowel disease. How much does her owner want to do in terms of testing at this time? This is a conversation I would rather have in person.

As difficult as it can be to get information over the phone, in-person conversations are not always straightforward. People often have trouble remembering timelines, especially for chronic issues. A client may tell me the cough became worse only yesterday and, a few moments later, describe how the pet had kept her up at night over the previous weekend with his cough. As I tend to take notes during my conversation with the owner, my writings can become rather messy.

In school, I was trained to ask a battery of questions to try to understand the chronology of the patient's symptoms. But I soon found that I needed to understand more than just those questions to get a real view of my patient and their caretaker. I needed information that would give me a window into my patient's life: how they fit into their family, and what the client's expectations were.

If multiple family members were involved in my patient's care, they often disagreed, which drove me wild. Couples were the worst. I complained about this once to my father, who subsequently related a story about his time working with customs agents at an airport. He had designed a drug detector for use at airports and was present for some of the on-site testing.

"When a couple arrives at the airport from another country and they are questioned by a customs agent, they never agree with each other," my father explained. "They're tired and cranky and can't remember what they bought. A couple with the exact same story is a red flag for inspectors, because they've probably rehearsed what to say." This made me take a step back and realize that owners weren't trying to be difficult; they were just worried about the animals they loved.

A simple question about a sick pet—*How long has Josie been vomiting?*—can elicit a conversation like this:

Spouse A. Well, the vomiting started last week.

Spouse B. *What?* It's been at least three weeks. If not more than that.

Spouse A, *shaking head vigorously.* No, no, it only started after the holiday.

Spouse B. You don't remember because you aren't the one who cleans it up. I'm the one who steps in it, so I'm the one who cleans it. Which, by the way, we need to talk about—

Spouse A. Wait, I don't think it was Josie three weeks ago; it was Lucy who vomited, after she got into the trash, remember?

Spouse B. That was *months* ago! When your mother visited!

Me. Okay, um, any changes in Josie's diet?

Spouse A. Nope, not at all. She eats exactly the same thing she's eaten for years.

Spouse B. Except for that big bag of food the neighbors gave us after their cat died.

I do realize that I am not alone in this frustration; other professionals also struggle to get histories from their patients and clients. Some years ago, I visited a physical therapist. During his initial consultation with me, he asked me to summarize my history of chronic issues with my foot and shoulders. I gave a concise description and timeline of my issues, flare-ups, treatments, and responses. After I finished, the physical therapist looked at me in surprise.

"That," he said, "was the *best* medical summary I have ever heard."

People often ask me, "How do you know what's wrong with your patients when they don't talk?"

The fact that my patients cannot speak is not something I think about; perhaps it is something I would consider if I had practiced first on humans and then switched to animals, but I have never treated patients who could communicate through written or spoken language. I've always had to deduce, detect, and read between the lines.

I imagine it might be like working as a pediatrician. You learn which questions to ask of the caretakers, and you learn to interpret the body language of your patients. It is also vitally important to perform a thorough physical exam. If I wonder whether the abdomen is painful, I'll palpate the area as I watch the animal closely for signs of discomfort and as my hands feel for tension in the muscles. I'll ask the client for their opinion and try to gain as much information as I can from their descriptions. *Gabriella cried when you picked her up? How were you holding her, exactly? Where did you put your hands?*

Veterinary medicine is a tactile occupation. I touch my patient, I draw up medication or vaccinations with a syringe, I write my notes. I love the phrase *the laying on of hands*, which always brings to mind my grandfather's gentle touch. When I looked up the phrase, I learned it has a religious meaning, yet to me it has always seemed a perfect phrase to describe the physical exam given by a doctor. The touching of another being with intent to help, and to convey a message: *I care.*

My laying on of hands is not always welcome by my patients. If anything, I am surprised by how many animals allow me to touch them, as relatively few dogs and cats try to bite or scratch. Most of the time, when a dog first tries to bite, their intention is to warn, not to harm. I know this because there have been many times I

have felt teeth on my hands but not been injured. During a veterinary exam or procedure, many dogs will growl or give another first
warning like lift a lip in the beginnings of a snarl, and others won't,
although you can tell from their body language that they are not
happy. Some may whine and shake. Yet most dogs will nip instead
of bite, and don't break the skin. I am so grateful to all the dogs who
choose not to harm me.

Then there are the dogs who mean to bite you the first time, with
no other warning. These, along with dogs who are termed "fear aggressive" and will attack first out of fear, are the most dangerous
types of canine patients. In the clinic, we write CAUTION or WILL
BITE in big letters on the chart as a heads-up: *this dog is potentially
dangerous and may give a serious bite with no warning.*

Cats are completely different. Although most are easy to handle,
if they do bite or scratch, they tend to be serious the first time.
There are some cats I can do anything at all to—for about thirty
seconds. Then, with no warning, the previously docile animal will
explode into a writhing, growling, furry ball of teeth and claws.
Some cats will growl but are mostly "talk," yet I tend to give them
the benefit of the doubt. And although it's dogs who are said to
be able to bond with one individual, I have met many one-person
cats—cats tightly bonded to one family member, who is able to
hold them, and calm them, while no one else can.

I realized early on that if I was rushed or distracted, I was more
likely to be injured by a patient, but if I was focused, I could better
read my patient and adjust to their reactions. Years later, I realized
that the focused state had a name: mindfulness. My work was actually safer if I was mindful and "in the moment." It made me a better
doctor, too.

I also tried to tune into my intuition. If a certain look in a dog's
eyes made me hesitate, even though the owner assured me the dog
had never bitten before, I knew I needed to use a muzzle, ask an as-

sistant for help, or even abandon the effort and make another plan. The times I ignored my judgment and forged on ahead were the times I'd get injured. I was learning to trust myself.

As a new graduate, I worried a lot about my patients. This was partly due to my lack of experience and confidence; I was concerned I wasn't doing enough for them, had overlooked some vital part of their diagnosis, or hadn't thought of a medication that might help. I conscientiously tried to think of anything that could help them, discussing cases with colleagues and, late into the night, paging through books. As I gained experience, I realized I was increasingly looking things up for confirmation.

When a sick animal was hospitalized, I took the case especially to heart, concerned that my own shortcomings could cause me to overlook something that might contribute to my patient's illness or even demise.

One day, during my second year in practice, I was obsessively worrying over a hospitalized cat. That day, a veterinary assistant named Jennifer was in the treatment room with me, and she regarded me curiously. She was a high school student who had worked at the clinic for a few years and seen many animals come and go. The practice was in a rural community, and although many clients brought in well-loved and cared-for pets, people occasionally commented "It's just a cat"—something I rarely hear nowadays.

As I mulled over this sick cat's condition, Jennifer shrugged and said, "The cat's going to die anyway."

My first thought was *Wow, that is so callous*. A few minutes later, though, a realization struck me: *She's probably right!* As I considered the offhand comment, I realized that, most likely, no matter what I did or didn't do, this cat—along with many of my seriously ill patients—may very well "die anyway." I would still do my best, but

Jennifer's comment helped me realize there should be a limit on the pressure I put on myself and that the death of a patient does not necessarily represent a failure on my part.

Obviously, success meant fixing a medical problem. Yet all my patients had a potential life span far shorter than my own. If death meant failure, perhaps I was setting myself up to fail. Perhaps I needed a new way to judge my work.

I didn't yet know what that was, but over the years I would come to understand it.

Clinic practice also meant handling euthanasia appointments. Along with the practical matter of administering the injection and keeping the patient comfortable, I had to guide the client through the process, and learn to be comfortable around grief and intense emotions. I often felt like I didn't belong in the sacred space between human and animal at such a pivotal moment. It was a lot to get used to.

One day at the clinic, I picked up the next patient's file to discover that it was a euthanasia appointment. I looked at the medical record; the dog was very old and had been ill for some time, so it was a case where the client's decision, though difficult, appeared clear. I would not need to talk this owner through the decision-making process, so the procedure should be fairly straightforward.

I called them into the exam room and a tall, dark-haired woman entered, wearing sunglasses and carrying a small, ancient, scruffy black dog wrapped in a blanket. I saw tears on the woman's face.

"I'm so sorry," I murmured after introducing myself.

The woman nodded in response, and gently eased the dog, still wrapped in the blanket, onto the exam table.

"Be careful," she warned me. "You should put a muzzle on her in case she bites."

I thanked her for letting me know.

"She even bites *me*," she continued, her face crumpling. The pitch of her voice grew higher. "She's really a bitch, but I love her."

I looked at them: the blanket-covered, broken-down dog; the tearstained woman with a declaration of love. Both were strangers to me; yet in a few moments, I had grasped the depth of their relationship, and it was breathtaking.

In veterinary school, mixed in among the large courses such as anatomy, physiology, biochemistry, and cardiology, and the smaller courses such as pathology and embryology, was a little course called the Human-Animal Bond. We considered it a "fluff" class, and my friends and I surreptitiously exchanged notes as we learned about research showing the heart rates of test subjects decreasing as they patted their pets, and the synchronization evident in the bodies of people and animals sleeping on the same bed. *That's cool*, I thought, *but of course people love their pets.*

As a practicing veterinarian, the little fluff class was becoming far more relevant than I could have imagined. The human-animal bond would guide every decision my clients made about my patients—and it could pierce my soul with its simplicity and strength.

I have long forgotten the woman's name, and the dog's name, but those words—*She's really a bitch, but I love her*—have stayed with me. To me, they are a precise definition of unconditional love, and of family.

The pair helped me understand that people accept their pets wholeheartedly, just as they accept us. Where I saw a snarly old dog, the woman may have seen the bright eyes and licking tongue of the happy puppy she once was. She may have seen the little dog in her prime: running, playing, curled up asleep.

Then again, maybe she saw only the grumpy, tired old dog on the table.

Her dog.

At the beginning of a relationship with an animal, there may be much joy and the promise of shared experiences to come. I share in this delight when I see a new puppy or kitten patient or a newly adopted adult animal. When a beloved pet dies, I was learning, it marks not only the end of the physical relationship but also a turning point. All the shared affection and experiences are compounded. Then, the relationship is not a promise but a shimmering, multilayered, multicolored entity: it is love, fully realized.

I bear witness to the vast love possible between species, to the connections I have come to know as no less wondrous because they are common. Transcendent love between an animal and a person, I was beginning to realize, is as common as fur.

5

House Calls

My grandfather's example of part-time house calls and part-time clinic work had made a deep impression on me. So after a few years of full-time clinic work, I decided to give house calls a try. By then, I had given up my idea of international work. I knew I didn't want to leave Trudy and Daiquiri for extended periods or find them a new home so I could work overseas. And I really enjoyed working with dogs and cats. I especially loved the opportunity to witness the bonds between human and animal that I got to see every day. Working in people's homes would bring me even closer to these unique relationships.

I'll give it a year, I reasoned. That should be long enough to decide whether house calls were for me. I obtained a part-time job at a different clinic nearby and went about setting up my own tiny practice. Although it was not nearly as complicated as opening a brick-and-mortar practice, I was still nervous. It seemed like an enormous responsibility, but Oupa's example gave me courage. I named my business Fine Veterinary House Calls.

I retrieved my grandfather's briefcase-style doctor bag from the closet, opening the various compartments as I ran my hands over the case. The medical instruments were still inside, as well as a battery-operated ophthalmoscope and otoscope unit that still worked. Despite the differences in species, countries, and era of our respective medical practices, the bag would work as a veterinary house-call bag. By ordering a new head for the scope I was able to use it as well, looking into the eyes and ears of my patients with my hand where my grandfather's had been.

I ordered supplies, setting up accounts with veterinary distributors to stock vaccinations, syringes, and basic medications, including pills to prevent heartworm disease and flea and tick products. I needed a centrifuge to "spin" the blood I drew before it was sent to the diagnostic lab, which would pick up samples from my house. I brainstormed with Karen, who had moved to Maine, about what else I would need.

"A microscope? To look at fecal and urine samples?" she suggested.

"Hmm. If I had a utility sink, maybe. I just can't see using my kitchen or bathroom sink. I'll have to send them out to the lab and pay the lab to run them."

"Let's see, you'll need blood tubes, a tourniquet, glass slides, urine cups, bandage materials, ear medications, eye medications, antibiotics, prescription labels, prescription pads, reminder cards, gloves . . ."

The list seemed endless.

At an appliance store, I chose a small dorm-sized fridge in which to store my vaccines.

"The freezer part doesn't work so well in these little ones," the salesman pointed out. "So you wouldn't want to put ice cream in it."

"That's okay, I'm not going to use it for food," I responded.

He frowned in confusion, but I was already on my way to the cashier.

I had recently moved to a small house on a lake that had a spare bedroom I could use as an office. I set up a business phone line, a fax machine, and a separate bank account. I ordered client folders, receipts, and rabies tags and certificates. I registered my business with the city, and with the state to collect sales tax. I purchased an ad in the Yellow Pages, where people used to look up things before the Internet, and printed some flyers to hang up at pet supply stores. I knew all the work I was doing was simple compared to setting up a clinic—which I couldn't have afforded to do, even if I'd wanted to. I would have needed to hire staff and purchase surgical equipment, anesthesia machines, an X-ray machine and table, machines to run in-house blood tests, cages for hospitalized animals, and enough pharmaceuticals to stock a clinic pharmacy. In comparison, setting up a house-call practice was easy.

Almost immediately, I knew I had found my niche. The benefits of a house-call practice included a flexible schedule, a slower pace, and working out of a home office. Most of my clients were quite appreciative, as I was often making their lives easier. Working part-time at the clinic helped me to not feel isolated professionally and allowed me to continue to perform surgery and interpret X-rays.

The downsides of my new career included no paid sick or vacation time and handling all my own appointments and paperwork.

The house-call life is somewhat mysterious to a "regular" veterinarian working in a clinic full-time. Another veterinarian once asked me whether all my patients were pampered house pets, summoning images of immaculately groomed cats lounging on velvet pillows. I laughed. The truth is my clients tend to be regular people who really love their pets. Some have multiple animals, some have dogs or cats that panic at the veterinarian's office or during the car ride, some are elderly or disabled people who do not drive, and others simply prefer the more involved, intimate relationship that comes with having a house-call veterinarian.

Going on house calls also allowed me the opportunity to see my patients in their home environment, and problem-solving sometimes became much simpler.

Peanut was a happy little shih tzu who was always excited to see me. His owner, a senior citizen, lived in a second-floor apartment, and she and Peanut liked to wait outside for me on their small, elevated deck. "Hi, Karen!" his owner, Jean, would call out in welcome as I got out of my car. Jean's voice was one I recognized when it played on my answering machine, and hearing it made me smile. Peanut always did a little dance of joy as I climbed the stairs.

Jean had trained Peanut to urinate on newspapers on the kitchen floor. One day, Jean called to tell me that Peanut was not urinating on his regular newspapers. This had never happened before, and we scheduled an appointment.

Although it was December, Peanut and Jean were waiting outside when I arrived. Peanut barked and spun in circles as I climbed the stairs. We entered the apartment, and I sat down in the kitchen in my usual chair. Before I bent down to retrieve Peanut's chart from my bag, I looked around, noticing that the apartment looked different.

Jean had decorated for Christmas, and wreaths, snowmen, and angels abounded. The area of the kitchen floor where Peanut's newspapers usually were was now occupied by an enormous planter, and the newspapers were moved to the side. The planter was larger than my patient.

I mentioned to Jean that perhaps her dog was intimidated by the change in his toilet surroundings. Jean and I moved the planter and replaced the newspapers, and Peanut immediately went over and urinated on them. I knew that had I seen Peanut at the clinic, it would have been much harder to realize what was causing the dog's behavior change.

————

I saw an elderly couple, Dick and Claire, who had a potbellied pig named Arnell. Arnell lived inside the house with them, and twice a year, she needed to have her nails trimmed and her ears cleaned. As she had grown too large to go in the car—well over one hundred pounds, too large for me to weigh—they asked for a house call. To hold the large pig down took three adults. After Dick became red-faced one day while holding her, I either brought helpers along or they recruited neighbors. Arnell's care was a group effort. Afterward, Dick and Claire served pizza and soda, and pressed a couple of twenty-dollar bills into my hand. I never officially charged them for her care.

It felt different, taking care of my patients in their homes. In a clinical setting, I was referred to as Dr. Fine, which seemed appropriate. I didn't know my clients well, and I preferred the formality, especially after working so hard to be taken seriously by clients and coworkers. In people's homes, however, there was a different level of familiarity. When I sat at a kitchen table or in a living room, I felt comfortable with clients calling me by my first name.

I would start each day by either answering the ringing phone or by finding a new message on my answering machine from someone wanting me to come out and check in on their pet. I did all my own scheduling (and answered my own phone), so after consulting with the caller for a few minutes, I would make arrangements to see their animal in between the appointments I already had scheduled. Where I could fit them in depended upon what town I was heading to as well as how urgent the animal's problem was. I liked that about my day. I liked that I never knew what it would bring. In that way, it was very different from the regimented life I'd had at the clinic, where appointments were scheduled every fifteen minutes. But it also meant I was always "on," which could be exhausting in a different way.

I would spend my days driving from home to home, whether

in the Massachusetts countryside or a city apartment, meeting animals, chatting with owners, drinking tea or sharing snacks, and moving on to the next appointment on my list. At lunchtime, I would head back home to do paperwork. I would do inventory, order new supplies, send out rabies certificates, and pay my bills. I would always try to make sure I was home in time for *All My Children*.

Old habits die hard.

Not long after owning ferrets became legal in Massachusetts, a young couple called me to come to their home to treat their ferrets. I was surprised that they'd used the plural as ferrets are generally smelly animals, and, like multiple cats using the same litter box, they could really stink up a house. I didn't know anyone with more than two. As part of the intake over the phone, I asked exactly how many ferrets I would be coming to see. "Ten," the woman said. "We have ten ferrets."

When I pulled up to the address they gave me, I grew especially concerned. This was not a large farmhouse, where l'eau de ferret might be spread over a large area. Rather, they lived in a condo, the sort that generally has about two or three bedrooms. In my time as a vet, I had encountered many smelly situations, and as I lifted my grandfather's medical bag off the passenger seat, I prepared for another one. I recalled the time I had noticed a strong odor from all the way outside on the doorstep of a house. It had turned out that my patient, a large dog, had been urinating on the shag rug in the living room for nearly a decade. I'd gone straight home and showered after that appointment.

Now this couple opened the door, and I braced myself. However, as I stepped inside, I smelled nothing. I walked with them through the condo and found that they kept the ferrets in their own gated alcove. It was a ferret paradise. It was filled with toys and hammocks that the ferrets lounged in adorably. All ten were rescues, and they all got along well and played together. That's when I checked my assumptions and got to examining the tiny creatures, one by one.

The ten-ferret household helped me realize the importance of being open-minded about what I might find when I encountered a new client. Each home was like a new world, and things sometimes looked and felt different there than they did in my own household or in the clinic. Years later, when I learned about narrative medicine, I realized that going into a home for the first time was like watching the beginning of a movie or reading the first pages of a book; I needed to acclimate myself to the surroundings to begin to understand the story of my patient.

I soon learned that cats needed to be corralled before my arrival, as most were smart enough to recognize that I was no ordinary guest. Kitties that were normally easygoing when visitors arrived suddenly relocated to hard-to-reach spots in basements, behind sofas, or underneath bed frames when the visitor was me. What ensued was a cat chase as the poor creature ran from secluded spot to secluded spot. If the client or I did manage to catch the cat, my patient was already stressed and anxious before I even started my exam. If we didn't catch the cat, I'd need to reschedule. As a result, I typically asked for people to confine even cooperative cats to a bathroom before I got there.

Once I arrived in the home, I'd get a history from the client just like I did at the clinic. I'd ask how the cat was doing, whether they went outdoors, what they ate. Then I'd get any vaccines ready and proceed to the bathroom with my stethoscope, scale, and chart.

If you want to get to know someone, try examining a cat in their bathroom. I found that some bathrooms were clean, and some were not. Also, some cats were amenable to being picked up, and some were not, in which case I knelt on the floor by the bathroom door, as cats often felt most comfortable near the exit, even if the door was closed. (After several years of bathroom-floor work, I was diagnosed with something called housemaid's knee, a painless swelling on my knees from extended kneeling on hard surfaces. I call it house vet's knee.)

Bonnie was a client with multiple pets, most of whom were easy to handle. One cat, a black-and-white kitty named Ming Fu, was difficult to catch, and had escaped during my last visit, missing her examination and the rabies vaccination required by law. At my next visit, I asked Bonnie to confine her to the bathroom before I arrived.

"She's always been a tough one," Bonnie warned me. I opened the bathroom door to find a large room with a laundry area and a long counter by the sink I could use as an exam table, saving my knees. I was able to pick up the nervous cat, perform an exam, and give her the required rabies vaccination. Just after the injection, though, she flew out of my hands, and I had no choice but to let her go. Unfortunately, she flew toward the toilet, and as I watched I realized in horror that the seat had been left up. Sure enough, Ming Fu splashed down right into the bowl. By now sopping wet and completely incensed, she leaped straight up and across the room, landed on top of the dryer, and disappeared behind it into the space between the machine and the wall.

I felt bad that she had gotten so stressed during my visit, but Bonnie just laughed. "Poor thing. Oh well, if she's all wet, maybe she'll act like a feather duster and clean out the space behind the dryer!" Bonnie was relieved that Ming Fu had been able to be vaccinated. We concluded that next time, we'd make sure the toilet lid was down.

It was surprising how often human toilets played a role in my work. Ebony was a short-haired black cat who was very difficult to catch, but her owner, Sharon, was able to confine her to the bathroom. It was a beautiful large bathroom with a sunken tub, but try as I could, I was unable to get near Ebony. Even though I approached her incredibly slowly, the cat always managed to keep a few feet of distance between us. After a good ten or fifteen minutes of this, I got tired and sat down on the closed toilet seat. I knew the next step was to use my fishing net, which I always tried to avoid. But as soon as I sat down, Ebony came right up to me. Of course, I realized, she was used to humans sitting on the toilet, and was much more comfortable with that behavior than with being stalked around the room by a stranger. She was clearly accustomed to being patted by Sharon while she used the bathroom. After petting Ebony for a minute or so, I was able to pick her up and give her a checkup with no issues. "Keep patting her when you're in the bathroom!" I advised Sharon before I left.

An elderly woman named Charlotte lived in a little apartment in the town's senior housing with her two cats. When we scheduled their annual checkup, she asked me for a favor. Her neighbor had a cat who also needed a checkup. Would I take care of her cat, too, without charging an additional house-call fee?

I told Charlotte that was no problem. This was something I did often for clients. When I arrived, however, I realized there'd been a misunderstanding. I'd assumed I would visit the neighbor in her own apartment, but the woman, along with her cat in a carrier, was sitting in Charlotte's tiny kitchen. Charlotte's cats were distressed by the unexpected visitor, as cats are often territorial and don't like intruders in their midst. The cat in the carrier was highly annoyed as well. It was not a good start to the visit.

The neighbor's cat was jumpy, and she tried to scratch me while I examined her. But I'd learned by then how to avoid being harmed. Or so I thought.

Once the neighbor's cat left, I focused on Charlotte's cats, who were usually friendly and easy to handle. Spunky, the male cat, proceeded as he normally did, no longer bothered by the noxious interloper. But Mochi was a different story. She was still agitated and would not let me get close to her. However, I knew Mochi. I knew that as soon as I picked her up, she'd be fine. I decided to use a soft leash as a lasso and impressed even myself when I managed to loop it around her neck.

However, Mochi was less impressed. She exploded. Charlotte's knickknacks, arranged so carefully on the shelves, went flying as Mochi tore around the small apartment trying to get rid of the thing on her neck. She came toward me and, instead of scurrying around me, climbed up me like a tree. She grabbed onto the back of my thigh with her sharp claws. I screamed.

Finally the leash came off, and Mochi disappeared into whatever nook she took comfort in. I sat in Charlotte's bathroom with a box of Band-Aids, taping them over the scratch marks all over my legs. By the time I emerged from the bathroom, Mochi had left her hiding place and was sitting calmly on a kitchen chair as if nothing had happened. I picked her up, examined her, and vaccinated her without further issue.

As I was leaving, Charlotte handed me a gift: a pretty candle, complete with a bow, to show her appreciation that I had been willing to see her neighbor's cat. I thanked her sheepishly and limped off to my car.

A year later, I stood at Charlotte's door again, cautiously optimistic. The little TV in her kitchen was on, and she beamed at it. "That nice Ellen finally got married," she said as she turned down the volume. We spoke about our mutual regard for the comedian and talk show host, then spent a moment reminiscing about the previous year's appointment. "I've never heard anyone *scream* like you did," she remarked. It made for quite a reputation. Fortunately

I managed to get through that visit without disturbing any knick-knacks or needing Band-Aids.

I first met Lisa when she called me about her cat, Mimi.

"I have an old cat, and last night, she was in my bed, and I still can't believe this, but she actually peed on my head!"

I waited for the next words, which I was afraid might be *So I need to make an appointment to have her euthanized.*

"So I need to make an appointment to have her checked out." Lisa laughed. I smiled in relief.

When I arrived for the appointment, Lisa and I hit it off right away. Her apartment was full of interesting books along with colorful artwork from around the world. We were the same age, we discovered. Lisa was an attorney working for a legal aid organization, advising people who couldn't afford to hire their own lawyer.

I examined Mimi, a sweet little tiger kitty, and drew a blood sample. After we finished, Lisa scheduled another appointment for me to check out her other pets. At that appointment, she invited me to stay for supper, and I was happy to accept. During dinner, we talked about books, and she invited me to join her book club. The friendship was sealed. Lisa later confessed to scheduling the appointment near dinnertime because she planned to invite me to dinner; I joked that she wanted me for a friend because of her many pets. Both of us recognized that the friendship, though new, would be a deep and lasting one.

Little Mimi turned out to have chronic renal failure (CRF). This is a common condition that affects older cats. While many cats with CRF live for years, some become uncomfortable relatively soon after the diagnosis, so the course of the disease can be hard to predict. Lisa sighed with resignation as I explained everything.

"She was old when I got her," she said, describing how she had adopted Mimi from a family member who couldn't keep her. "It seems like she's always been old."

Yet a few years passed and Mimi hung on. She was ancient and mostly incontinent; most of the time she slept. Lisa and her husband, Joe, were planning a three-month sabbatical in Mexico; they intended to drive there in their station wagon along with their two large dogs, camping along the way. Before they left, Lisa reluctantly decided it was time to schedule Mimi's euthanasia. Joe would be at the house by himself for the appointment, she explained, because he was a paramedic and didn't mind dealing with medical procedures. Lisa herself felt uncomfortable with the thought of being present when Mimi died. She wanted to remember Mimi as she was when she was alive. I understood; lots of people don't feel comfortable witnessing euthanasia procedures, and I never pressured someone to be present for the procedure if they didn't want to be there.

On the appointed day, I drove to Lisa's house. Lisa met me at the door with a broad smile. I was confused. Why was she home? And why was she smiling?

"Joe had a great idea!" Lisa proclaimed.

I glanced over at Joe, who was standing in the kitchen. His arms were folded and his lips compressed as he stared off into the middle distance. He did not look like a guy who'd had a great idea.

I turned back to Lisa. "Last night, I was crying and crying and crying about Mimi," my friend explained, the words tumbling out as they did when she was happy and excited about something. "And then Joe said, 'The only other option would be to bring her with us.' And I said, 'Yes, that's it! We'll bring her with us!'"

"Bring her with you?" I repeated.

"Sure! She's always been good in the car. We won't even know she's there."

"Camping?" I asked, trying to picture sleeping in a tent on a cross-country road trip with a frail, incontinent cat in addition to two large dogs. "Are you sure?"

"Of course!" said Lisa. "She'll be fine. It's the perfect solution!"

I looked over at Joe again. He was shaking his head in resignation. Lisa's mind was made up, we could tell. Little Mimi was going to Mexico.

I got to see it firsthand. Lisa and Joe invited me to visit them during their stay in Mexico, and I spent a wonderful week with them; we joked that it was my farthest house call. They had rented a small apartment near the beach in a little town. Mimi was a sweet little thing, light as a feather, and seemed happy to snooze in her little bed in the kitchen, enjoying her sabbatical.

Eventually Mimi and her humans traveled back to Worcester, the little cat at one time alarming Lisa by wandering some distance away from the car at a rest stop. She continued her routine of sleeping much of the day and urinated wherever she chose, but never again on Lisa's head.

Mimi surprised us all and lived for several more months before Lisa made the euthanasia decision again. This time, Mimi had stopped eating, and Lisa knew there would be no reprieve. The setup would be the same as we had discussed before: Joe would be at home alone when I arrived.

As I drove to Lisa and Joe's house for Mimi's second euthanasia appointment, I wondered whether the procedure would be different with a client I knew well who had a medical background. Joe had seen death before. He would take this in stride, I imagined. Also, Mimi had been more Lisa's cat than his.

Joe met me at the door, holding Mimi in his arms. His face was red and soaking wet. Tears dripped down both cheeks, which he made no attempt to wipe. His nose dripped, too, as he bent his head to kiss Mimi's soft fur.

"I didn't think I'd be this upset," he choked out.

"Oh, that's okay, of course that's okay," I said, giving him a quick hug.

"It's just . . . we've had her for so long." He gulped. "She's been such a good cat."

Mimi had been old ever since we had known her, and because she had lived for so long, it was hard to believe her time had finally arrived. She died peacefully, in Joe's arms, as we cried together. Joe and Lisa later planted a tree for her in their garden, to honor this little old cat who had gone on a sabbatical to Mexico and who brought my friend and me together.

Although I enjoyed home visits, running my own business was also scary. If I felt unable to handle something, I couldn't just ask another veterinarian in the practice or open a book at my desk. I was on my own, and I was not in control of the environment. I also worried about my personal safety. Most people who called me, it turned out, were women. It may have been irrational, but if a man called and mentioned a wife or girlfriend or if I suspected he was gay, I felt safer. Lisa offered to come with me if I ever needed backup, and I did take her up on it a few times.

I needed a way to lower my stress level, and I had heard that yoga could help, so I signed up for a beginner class at a nearby yoga center. There were different classes and different teachers, but I was fortunate to sign up with Ann Bissanti, a master yoga teacher who had trained in India with noted yoga teacher B. K. S. Iyengar. Ann's classes took her students deep into the connection between mind and body. I learned how to bring my mind back to the breath, over and over, and how to meditate within the pose. Yoga helped me so much that I couldn't imagine how I had lived without it. Even though I practiced only in class and not at home, I was less anxious.

If I missed a few classes, I could tell a difference; I didn't sleep as well and was quicker to anger, so I tried to make time for class even if I was unusually busy.

House calls allowed me to observe my patients' and clients' stories in greater depth, which helped me individualize their treatment. It also gave me a sense of community for the first time in my life. I had grown up so alone with so little around me in terms of family, I hadn't even known how much I'd been missing. Some clients invited me to stay for dinner or sent me home with gifts, and I recognized many of their voices when I heard them on my answering machine. Because I got to know both people and animals better from being in their homes, I came to feel like extended family to many of them. I belonged.

6

Where Puppies Come From

One day, I received a call from a pet store in a nearby town. Pet stores used to be easily recognizable; they were called pet stores and located in malls or shopping centers. This store was in a private home and called itself a kennel. They did breed a couple of types of dogs on-site, the owner told me, but most of their puppies were shipped to them from out of state. I knew these puppies were bred and sold as commodities, likely by puppy mills, where they were bred for profit in questionable conditions and shipped hundreds of miles in crowded trucks. The owner assured me their puppies were purchased from "reputable breeders," a term open to interpretation. I knew that no self-respecting breeder would sell their puppies to a pet store or broker who would then sell them to any random person with a credit card. This "kennel" was not the sort of business I wanted anything to do with.

"The law requires the puppies to be examined once a week," the owner told me. I'll call her Sandy. She and her husband were looking for a new veterinarian to come weekly—preferably on a Friday so the puppies could be sold that weekend—and examine the animals, as their previous vet was no longer available.

"I know your time is valuable," Sandy said, quoting me a generous price. It was tempting; I could certainly use the money. House calls were proving to be enjoyable but not profitable. And I loved puppies. Yet my interest lay in the bond between animal and human. I didn't want to take the person out of the equation. And I wanted nothing to do with puppy mills. So I politely declined.

However, Sandy was not giving up that easily, and I was inexperienced at saying no. She begged and pleaded until I finally agreed to come once or twice and try it out. What could that hurt, I imagined. Perhaps I could have a positive influence on the place by advocating for the puppies and making sure they were well cared for.

On the appointed day, I arrived at the kennel, a large home in a rural area. I went in through the customer entrance to find a bright, welcoming space decorated in farmhouse style with comfortable chairs, dog pictures on the walls, a large wooden desk, and a gated-off area in one corner where a young couple was looking at two puppies. I introduced myself to the teenage girl at the desk, who said she'd be with me in a moment. I turned to observe the two puppies in the gated area; while one played and acted normally, the other, a yellow Lab, looked lethargic and vomited some brown liquid as I watched.

"All set," said the girl, who introduced herself as Jen. I asked for Sandy, but Jen said that Sandy and her husband were away on vacation at the beach. I was surprised; Sandy had not mentioned on the phone that she wouldn't be present. Jen explained that she would bring me into the basement, where the puppies were housed and where clients were not allowed.

I followed Jen down a narrow staircase and through an equally narrow hallway. The basement had been subdivided into a warren of small rooms. There were no dog pictures or comfy chairs down here. The walls were not even visible, as each room was lined from floor to ceiling with rows of small cages, and the cages were filled with puppies. There didn't seem to be much ventilation, I noticed; the air was stuffy and the rooms smelled of puppy waste. Jen and I reached the end of the hallway, where a slightly larger room was set up for puppy treatments and exams.

"We'll bring them to you," Jen said. There were a few other teenagers around, and one of them showed me the paperwork on each puppy and what I would need to fill out and sign. I was shocked to note that my name had been preprinted on the business forms as the kennel veterinarian, although I had clearly told the owner I was not interested in a permanent position. It seemed they assumed I would continue.

As a veterinary professional, I needed to keep my own records, so I set up my chart.

Then the puppy parade began.

One pup at a time, the young staff brought me Labradors and Lhasa Apsos, Boston terriers and boxers, shih tzus and Saint Bernards. Yorkshire terriers. Samoyeds. Poodles, Pomeranians, border collies, and several other breeds. This was before the current craze of breed combinations and doodles, but it was still a large variety of dogs.

Each puppy was identified by an individual number, as well as what number room they were housed in. Some were healthy, but many seemed sickly, with thick yellow nasal discharge and weepy eyes. It was not something I typically saw when I examined puppies at the clinic. But these puppies had not been born on-site; they had been shipped from out of state, the stress of which could make them more vulnerable to infection. They were housed in cramped cages with little ventilation and had likely been transported in similar conditions. It was a rough start for any puppy. Add to that being born and spending their initial weeks of life in similar or worse conditions, and the possibility of inherited problems due to their parents not being screened for health or genetic conditions common within their particular breed . . . It was not a place where I would want to get a puppy.

I asked questions about the sick ones, just as I would have at the clinic or at someone's home: How long has this been going on? How are they acting? Have they had diarrhea? Have they coughed or vomited? Are they eating normally? The answer for each puppy was the same: the staff didn't know. It wasn't even written down anywhere. No one seemed to pay attention to the welfare of the individual animals. It was quite different from the litters of puppies I'd examined from real breeders who'd bred the dogs themselves. Good breeders, I knew, breed animals with a focus on good health and temperament, because they love the breed.* They ensure that both parents are friendly and social, and they don't breed dogs with medical problems. Good breeders are committed to their puppies and want them back if the owner can't keep them anymore. They know each puppy's personality and try to match it to the home the puppy is going to: an energetic pup to an active home, and a shy pup to a quiet home. Puppy mills don't care about any of that. They don't know the animals' temperaments and take no time to socialize them. It is only about the money.

The records for each animal listed the medications they were on, as required by law. Most of the pups that appeared healthy were either currently taking antibiotics or had just finished a course of antibiotics. The business was using a very strong antibiotic, one that veterinarians rarely use because it carries a slight risk to humans. People are supposed to wear gloves when administering this medi-

---

* See "How to Find a Good Breeder" on page 291–292 for more information on locating a reputable breeder.

cation to their pets. I asked Jen if the staff wore gloves when they gave the puppies medication and she looked at me blankly; clearly, they did not.

About an hour into the puppy exams, a man in uniform walked in and introduced himself as an officer from the MSPCA, the state's division of the Society for the Prevention of Cruelty to Animals. I was thrilled to see him and listed my concerns about the sick puppies, the lack of ventilation, and the overuse of antibiotics. He was not surprised.

"We're trying to work with them to improve things," he said, handing me his card. I put it in my pocket, thanked him, and got back to work. I examined puppies, wrote notes, and prescribed medications: antibiotics (different from the one they were using), ear medicines, and eye medicines. Many pups had dirty ears and what were likely ear mites.

As I got closer to finishing, the staff seemed progressively more anxious, exchanging nervous glances and whispering to one another.

"You know, any of them you prescribe medication for, we can't sell this weekend," Jen finally explained. "It's the state law. Sandy's not going to like this."

I looked at her in confusion. Apparently she expected me to not prescribe medication for the animals that I felt required it so they could be put up for sale the following day.

"If a puppy needs medication, I'm going to prescribe it," I said simply.

A few minutes later, one of the teenagers approached me with a cordless phone. "It's Sandy," she said.

I took the phone. Sandy was agitated and seemed close to tears as she begged me to reconsider. But this time, I was not going to give in. As well as the health of the puppies, my veterinary license was at stake. Sandy's weekend puppy sale prospects could not be a part of my decision-making.

It was a tense conversation. I could tell I would not be welcomed back as their regular veterinarian even if I wanted to return. I was glad Sandy was away, as I'm sure the dispute would have been even worse in person.

When I finally finished, I had examined eighty-seven puppies. The number of puppies in the basement was akin to a hoarding situation that might qualify as a leading news story, except this was a licensed business. These puppies would not be released to shelters that would nurse them to better health and make sure they went to good homes, ones that were a good fit for them as individuals. Instead, they were sold for profit as is, with a "health guarantee" that many buyers don't realize typically means only that the business will exchange a sick puppy for a healthy one, not pay for any veterinary care.

The mood was somber as Jen filled out the check pre-signed by Sandy, who called back as I was walking out the front door. No, I told her firmly, I was not going to reconsider.

I got into my car and decided to do something I'd never done before: I went straight to the bank the check was written from, in the town center, and cashed the check. I was worried that Sandy would cancel the check before I could deposit it. I had worked hard for the money and done my best for those puppies. I hoped the next veterinarian they hired would likewise advocate for their care.

Still, I couldn't get the puppies and the stuffy overcrowded basement out of my mind. Maybe I could have held off prescribing medications for some of those puppies with ear problems, I thought. Then they could have left the overcrowded basement sooner and hopefully gone to new homes. But that, I reminded myself, would only make room for new truckloads of puppies to be delivered the following week.

Sandy and the other people contributing to the puppy mill trade probably had nothing against puppies. They simply saw them as commodities, not individual beings. They knew many people want a puppy right away and don't want to research reputable local breeders or wait until a litter is born. Some people also assume that shelter animals have poor health or temperaments, not realizing the animals are often far better cared for, socialized, and evaluated than puppy mill puppies. Even a backyard breeder, a local person who decides to breed their (possibly puppy mill–acquired) dog, can potentially have advantages over a pet store, as the litter may be raised in a home instead of in a cage, socialized with people and children, and have the mother on-site to be met by potential puppy buyers.

People selling puppy mill puppies didn't care whether the buyers had previous experience with dogs or whether the pup's temperament would match their family. They weren't concerned, as I was, about whether a pup would go into a good home or end up as a stray, unclaimed, at a kill shelter. They also didn't encourage buyers to spay or neuter their pet to prevent unwanted litters of puppies that may also end up at a shelter. My concern came from personal experience. At the clinic where I worked, shelter dogs who had been unclaimed for ten days were brought in for the veterinarian to euthanize. These dogs were typically young adult mix-breed males, rambunctious and untrained. They exuded health and energy. They were often friendly, and sometimes tried to lick me through the muzzle placed on them by the animal control officer. Sometimes, if I thought a dog could be accepted by a no-kill shelter, I'd set the syringe with the bright pink liquid down on the counter.

"Let me see if I can place this one," I'd offer.

This involved several phone calls on my part. If I was lucky, I'd find a rescue to take in the dog. I'd then bring the dog home overnight and to the shelter the following day. I talked to Lisa a little bit about the stray dogs I saved. Like me, all her pets were rescues, and she was committed to saving lives.

The ones I didn't save, I didn't talk to anyone about.

I couldn't stop thinking about the puppies in Sandy's base-ment. Finally, I composed a formal letter to her, with a copy to the MSPCA officer. I didn't like to make enemies, but I felt I owed it to the puppies. I recommended better hygiene and ventilation for the facility and explained that the overwhelming antibiotic use should not be necessary and could contribute to antibiotic resistance. I rec-ommended identifying any sick puppies earlier and isolating them to prevent the spread of disease.

I imagined Sandy creating a voodoo doll in my image, stick-ing pins in me as she lamented her lost income. Well, at least she wouldn't be calling to pressure me to be their veterinarian again.

I wish I could say things have changed since I visited Sandy's kennel years ago. But they haven't. The laws continue to require only the most-basic care for dogs bred and sold as commodities; they are treated like livestock. The nonprofit Bailing Out Benji tracks large-scale breeding operations on its website, and many such businesses house dozens or even hundreds of adult dogs. I encourage clients and friends considering getting a puppy to check out shelters and rescues, read the American Humane Society web-site's puppy mill information, research local breed clubs for breeder recommendations, and check out journalist Rory Kress's excellent book *The Doggie in the Window*. But people aren't always patient when it comes to adopting a puppy, and it can be tempting to be-lieve what the Humane Society calls "puppy mill doublespeak" when faced with an adorable puppy. Some people even convince themselves they are rescuing the animal in question.

Many puppy mills have expanded their reach by becoming savvy marketers, and it's common for them to design flashy websites and to sell and ship their wares directly to the consumer, thus pocket-ing all the money. Online puppy broker sites are today's pet shops, and they know exactly what to say; they claim to abhor puppy mills and describe their puppies as "family-raised" by "reputable" breeders that meet strict criteria. Yet when I look at photos and videos of available pups, I see mostly confused, anxious animals who have been staged for pretty photo ops but do not appear well socialized. They look different from the happy, relaxed puppies on the Petfinder and Shelter Pet Project websites, which allow users to search shelters and rescues by location, age, and breed.[†]

One day at the clinic, I had an appointment with a sickly looking boxer puppy that the owner had picked up the previous day at the airport in Boston. The puppy was dehydrated and lethargic with a crusty nasal discharge, much like the puppies at Sandy's kennel.

"This isn't even the puppy I bought," said the owner.

I looked at her in surprise.

"I picked out the puppy I wanted from the website," the young woman explained. She pulled out her phone and showed me a picture. It was clearly a professional website, and the puppies were photographed on a grassy lawn. It was obvious that the pup on the table was not the one in the picture, as their markings were completely different. "The breeder always answered my calls before I paid, but now I can't get ahold of them, and they aren't calling me back," she said tearfully. "I mean, what am I going to do, send her back? I can't do that. Who knows what they would do? Put her to sleep, maybe." I could not disagree with her. And it was too late to explain that, as far as I was concerned, unless she had been to the breeder's home and met the pup's mother, the "reputable breeder" she had corresponded with was actually a puppy mill.

I know many of my dog patients come from puppy mills. Some have chronic health issues and behavior problems. Yet they are still dogs; they don't blame us for their origins, and they still bond to their people. Most of my patients are fortunate to have landed in loving homes where they are well cared for, but I still feel bad about

---

[†]   For a list of pet adoption agencies, see "Finding a New Pet" on page 291.

the rough start they had and for their parents, who are doomed to years of puppy mill life. The few dogs I've seen that have been adopted after being used as this kind of breeding stock had never before entered a house or played on grass. Puppy mill breeding animals are doomed to a life spent in a cage, unloved, their own medical issues untreated, as their worth is only in their ability to produce offspring. It's a poor way to care for the families of our beloved pets.

7

New Beginnings

Even when I wasn't examining puppies at a pet store, I saw lots of puppies at work. Puppies have always set off bells and whistles in my brain. Karen was a "baby person" and if she and I were out somewhere and saw a baby in a stroller, she'd ooh and aah, but I didn't see much to get excited about. Kittens were admittedly cute, but *puppies* . . . puppies melted my heart. Driving down the street, I'd stop my car if I saw one.

I knew Trudy wouldn't live forever, and I was worried about how I would handle her eventual loss. I had a vague idea about getting a puppy at some point in the next few years. Yet with all the puppies I saw, I needed to maintain an emotional distance and not allow myself to get attached, even to litters of puppies that were brought in for vaccines.

I was driving to work one morning when I glimpsed a brown-and-black dog by the side of the road in an unsettled area. I pulled over, got out of my car, and approached the animal, careful not to get too close. It was a puppy, I realized, and when I spoke encouragingly to him in a high-pitched tone he approached me, wagging his tail.

There were no houses nearby; how had this little one come to be there? Perhaps he'd run off and was a long way from home, or perhaps he'd been dumped. I hated to think of the possibility. At the clinic, I called the town's dog officer while we settled him into a cage. He had large paws and was going to be a big dog. I brought him home that night, calling him Boris. He was adorable and I was tempted to keep him, but he looked like he was going to be even larger than Trudy, and I wasn't quite ready to add to my family. Back at the clinic, we set up a kennel for him behind the front desk with a big sign that read FOR ADOPTION. No one called to claim him. But soon, a woman bringing her dog in for a checkup fell in love with him, and he went to a wonderful new home.

The day my emotional distance dissolved began like any other day. It had been a couple of years since I'd found Boris, and I was working at a different clinic. I was between appointments one morning when I saw a shelter worker named Amy enter the clinic by the side door, carrying a fawn-colored puppy with an injured paw. She explained that according to witnesses, the pup had been hit by not one, but two cars. When I saw the little ears flopping in Amy's arms, something changed inside me.

The puppy had short fur, dark eyebrows, and a dark muzzle, as though she had dipped her nose in paint. She also had two different-colored eyes, one brown and one a light sky blue, like a Siberian husky. Her tail curled upward. As I examined the wounded paw, she covered my hands with soft puppy kisses, and I felt an almost electric connection to the little being. In that instant, I knew with absolute certainty that I needed this puppy in my life. Fortunately, the pup, who was about three months old, had escaped with only a couple broken toes. I told Amy that I would bring her home, ostensibly to care for her injured paw, and that I wanted to keep her. Amy was thrilled, as she said that no one had called to claim her. After I examined the puppy, we settled her into a cage in the hospital area, where I caught her sleeping with her head in her partially tipped-over water bowl.

The rest of the day, I felt like I was floating. I knew my life had irreversibly changed. At one point, my logical mind intervened, reminding me that a puppy was an enormous commitment, and it was not in my nature to make such a big decision spontaneously. "This is crazy. I can't bring this puppy home," I told myself. I imagined *not* bringing her home. Immediately I was struck by a feeling of something being terribly wrong. I banished the thought.

I named my new dog Rana, short for Prana, which I knew from my yoga classes meant "life force energy" in Sanskrit. The little puppy seemed to have it in spades.

Little Rana turned out to be an outside-the-box thinker. She was very different from Trudy, who loved routine and always made sure she kept me in sight when we were in the woods. Rana loved to run off leash and sought out giant branches to carry, often getting stuck between trees. She also loved to swim, hurtling off the dock after a tennis ball with her legs splayed out at wild angles, so different from Trudy's precise dives. In the water, Rana chased after ducks, and each time they would swim away and eventually take flight, Rana would give one last burst of energy. Her little shoulders would rise out of the water as if she too might fly. Only after the ducks flew off would she turn around and head for home.

I've known many excellent pet owners who have had a dog or cat escape from a yard or house and run onto or across a road. All it takes is one slip of the collar or one unthinking guest or family member to leave a gate or a door open. Fortunately, most of the time the animal is recovered without incident, in what the airline industries term a "near miss." All my animals have had a near miss at one time or another, and if it can happen to a pet belonging to an overly cautious (some might say neurotic) veterinarian, then it can happen to anyone's pet.

One fall day, Trudy, then ten years old, and Rana, who was about ten months old, were out in the fenced backyard. When I went to call them in, I found only Trudy, who seemed confused.

The small yard was fenced, but a few areas were patched with chicken wire, and Rana had apparently wedged her way in between a connection and gotten loose.

My joyous free spirit of a dog was gone.

I was frantic. I grabbed some dog treats and ran around calling for her, but she had disappeared. I took Trudy out on leash, thinking maybe she would track Rana, but Trudy didn't drag me in any specific direction, so I brought her back home. I called the city dog officer, who said he would let me know if he heard anything. My little lake house was on a main road, with railroad tracks behind the houses across the street. I kept thinking: *The road, the lake, the train tracks. The road, the lake, the train tracks.* After running around my neighbors' houses and across the street yelling for Rana, I took to my car, desperate to find her and hoping she hadn't been hit by a car again.

I questioned any person I saw—*Did you see a tan-colored dog run by? Have you seen my dog? My dog is lost!* Everyone I spoke to was sympathetic, but no one had seen her. I kept driving and looking, driving and looking. An hour went by, but it felt like much longer. It seemed as though Rana had evaporated. *Where could she have gone?* I kept asking myself. I drove around in a frenzy, thinking I now understood the expression *I was beside myself.* I felt as though there were literally two of me: the real one driving and the frantic one inside me thinking that this could not be happening.

My cell phone rang. The city dog officer told me he had received a phone call from one of the valets at the nearby hospital, saying he had found a stray dog. The dog officer did not have a description of the dog. I drove straight to the hospital, two miles down the road and across a busy highway. Could Rana have gone this far, I wondered, and crossed this road? I screeched my car to a stop near the valet station and put my hazard lights on. There were several valets standing around near the booth by the hospital entrance. I don't know what they thought of me as I charged toward them, calling out, "My dog! Did one of you find my dog?"

"Rocky found a dog—he put it in his truck," one of the valets responded. "He's gone to get a car, but he'll be back in a minute."

"What does the dog . . . look like?" I panted, desperate to know whether it was Rana.

"Uh, I think it has two different-color eyes," he answered.

"Oh my God! That's her! It's her!" I felt a swell of relief. It had to be her!

Rocky, a tall blond teenager, arrived and led me to his truck while he explained what had happened. He had seen a dog running in and out of traffic and recognized she was likely to be hit by a car. He called to the dog and she came to him readily. He then put her in the back of his own vehicle and called the phone number on the dog license attached to her collar.

When I saw Rana's blue and brown eyes peeking out at me from the back of Rocky's truck, I burst into tears. I put my hand into my pocket and pulled out whatever money I happened to have in there, pressing the bills into Rocky's palm despite his embarrassed protestations. Hands trembling, I fastened Rana's leash, then hugged and touched her all over, checking her body for injuries.

My puppy had run for over two miles and crossed at least six lanes of traffic on a divided highway, yet she did not have a scratch on her.

The next day, I called Rocky's boss, wanting to make sure he did not get into trouble for taking time away from his work to save my dog. His boss assured me Rocky was not in trouble.

I felt as though Rocky had saved my life, not just Rana's; I was so grateful and happy that I felt an impulse to do something extravagant. I ordered several large pizzas to be delivered to the valets at lunchtime, and attached a card to one of the boxes, addressed to Rocky. Inside the card, I wrote, *Thank you so much for saving my puppy. Without you she would have been road pizza!*

My feeling of euphoria lasted a good two weeks. By then, a new and sturdy fence had been installed in my backyard. I began calling Rana "Rana T." because Trouble was her middle name.

Years later, I still think of Rocky every time I am driving and see a loose dog, and I stop my car or turn around and go back to look for them. Each time, I remind myself that once, someone stopped what they were doing, and went out of their way to save Rana. The rescue of a stray dog, whether it has a home or needs a home, can change many lives.

Rana's adoption left me open to other unexpected experiences. One day I was reading the newspaper and scanned the personal ads just for fun. One stood out to me. I answered it, something I had never done before. I couldn't believe I was actually replying—and to someone who shared the same name as my brother. But responding to the ad, I felt something of the same intuition I'd felt when I first saw Rana.

Mike was an environmental engineer whose passion for the environment was similar to my love for animals. He had a droll sense of humor and loved spending time in the woods. On one of our first dates, we went to see the movie *Best in Show*, a comedy about the dysfunctional people and (mostly) normal dogs involved in the dog show world.

"I am *not* like those people!" I insisted.

Mike smiled but refrained from commenting. He had heard the story about the pizza delivery for the valets.

We'd been on only a couple dates when Mike confessed to being dog phobic. He had been chased by neighborhood dogs as a young child and hadn't had much of a relationship with the family dogs of his childhood (spaniels his father kept for hunting pheasants). Despite his nervousness, I was impressed that he understood how important my pets were to me. Still, I had to make one thing clear.

I told him I was always going to have pets—especially dogs—in my life. Having grown up without them, I never wanted to be dog-less again. A long-term relationship with me meant agreeing to a life shared with dogs and cats. If he couldn't handle that, then we should end this before it went any further.

As Mike got to know Trudy, Rana, and Daiquiri, he warmed to them, buying them toys, caring for them if I was away, remarking on their quirks and habits. He even sang them silly little songs with me. In time, he would grow to love them.

I knew Mike was well on his way to becoming an animal person when he described an incident that occurred at his parents' house. He and his parents and sisters were looking at a book of photographs, one of which showed a harness-wearing working dog. "Awww," Mike exclaimed upon seeing the picture. His family members all turned to stare at him in surprise. None of them had ever heard him say "aw" about an animal before.

Mike was spending more and more time at my house, hanging out with me and the pets, enjoying the lake. One day I called him just as he was leaving to come over.

"Oh good, I'm glad I caught you. I'm going to make cookies and I'm not sure I have enough flour. Can you please bring some flour from your house?"

"I don't have flour," he responded. "I never buy flour."

"No *flour*? What if you want to make cookies?"

"I don't make cookies."

"Oh . . . okay. See you soon then." As a lifelong chocolate fiend, I always made sure I had chocolate chip cookie–making ingredients on hand. Mike, however, in addition to not being a baker, was a minimalist. Perhaps it stemmed from his enjoyment of backpacking, but he tended to have only the bare necessities around him. The fridge at his condo was so empty, he kept full jugs of water inside to help keep the temperature cool.

An avid hiker, Mike adapted to hiking with dogs, and I adapted to more time in the woods. If we weren't near other people, I'd usually let the dogs off leash. Trudy stayed right with us on the trail, but Rana was always taking off and crashing through bushes. It was hard to tell where she was, and I worried about losing her, but Mike thought of a solution. He bought Rana a cowbell, a heavy bell that we attached to her collar only when we were in the woods. Then we could tell where she was and keep track of her.

Mike gradually slid into the role of pet co-parent. One day he made a list of all the names and nicknames I had for each of the pets. Troodles was his favorite for Trudy. He enjoyed seeing how the names morphed into each other and Troodles became Strudel. He even started coming up with his own names for them. One day after I arrived home from work late, he said, "I fed the petlings," coining a term we continued to use for our animals.

Slowly, we met each other's families. Mike had four siblings, and three of them lived close by, as did his parents. His family welcomed me warmly. My parents had divorced after I graduated from veterinary school; my mother relocated to California, and my brother was living in Utah. My father stayed in Massachusetts and remarried.

My stepmother, Angela, was a dog person, and she had brought her aging spaniel, Molly, into the relationship. Angela and my father soon adopted another dog, a spaniel-mix puppy they named Petey. On one of Mike's first visits to their home, Petey ended up getting loose outside, and we all ran into the backyard woods to search for him. Finally I heard someone yell, "I've got him!"

It was Mike. I knew my father and Angela would have liked Mike anyway, but it didn't hurt that my dog-phobic boyfriend had rescued their new puppy.

We planned our first vacation together for the second week in September of 2001. Mike preferred vacationing in September because he liked the weather and the lack of crowds, and I liked it because I got a break from itchy dogs and cats during flea season. Mike wanted to visit a remote lake camp in northern Maine. I agreed to stay in a cabin with an outhouse, but I drew the line at eating canned food for the week. The camp offered a dinner option, so we signed up for home-cooked meals for most of the nights.

On the Tuesday morning of our trip, we packed a picnic lunch and canoed out to a trail where we hiked and picnicked. When it came time to canoe home, however, the wind had picked up and we were unable to canoe back against the strong current. Fortunately, there was a path along the lake, so we dragged the canoe to a dry spot and hiked back to camp, arriving midafternoon. We felt bad about abandoning the canoe and went in search of the camp owners to apologize and let them know we would retrieve it the following day. When we found one of the owners, she seemed dazed and kept talking about airplanes and buildings. She didn't care about the canoe. It was hard for Mike and me to comprehend what she was saying; it was almost as though she were speaking another language. When we finally realized what had happened, I borrowed the camp phone to call relatives and make sure they were okay as our cell phones did not have service. The camp didn't have a television, so all we learned about 9/11 in those first few days was from newspapers the camp owners brought back from town (an hour-long ride on dirt roads) and the shortwave radio I'd brought.

When we departed the camp on Saturday for the long drive home, it felt like we were entering a different world than the one we'd left a week earlier. American flags were everywhere, and signs on restaurants and buildings that had advertised sales and specials now held heartfelt messages like *God Bless America*. An armory we drove by was packed with army vehicles. Once we arrived home and turned on the television, I was glad Mike had chosen such a remote place. We had been spared the visuals that we would have been glued to had we been anywhere else.

The trip had drawn us together in ways we couldn't have imagined when we planned it. Mike even admitted to missing the petlings while we were away.

8

A Whole New Toolshed

It was easy to get to know my house-call clients as I sat in their homes and discussed their pets' health. But I also got to know some clients at the clinic where I worked part-time. One was a woman named Carol, who had a long-haired black cat named Smokey. Carol was a devoted cat owner and took fastidious care of her multiple cats. Normally I would have seen each cat only once a year for a checkup. Smokey, however, had chronic health problems, so I got to know him and Carol well.

Smokey had severe chronic inflammation of the inside of his mouth and throat, a challenging condition to manage. I'd treat it with a long-acting steroid injection, but it would just come back a month or two later. We tried changing his diet. We tried allergy medications. We tried antibiotics. Carol could not afford a referral to a specialist or putting Smokey under anesthesia to get a biopsy of the area. The injections worked well, so we continued with them, trying to make them as infrequent as possible.

As often as I saw Carol about Smokey, she never complained. Some people who had animals with chronic problems blamed the veterinarian. "I've had him in here three times for the same problem, and he's still not fixed!" Carol understood that I was doing my best for her cat and that feline health is as complex as human health. I tried to keep the recheck charges to a minimum so her costs were manageable. She was a pleasure to work with, as was Smokey.

One day, Carol brought Smokey in for a different problem. He was drinking and urinating a lot. We ran some blood tests, and I diagnosed Smokey with diabetes. I knew it was possible the multiple steroid injections had contributed to his diabetes. I felt bad about it, but Carol was serene, without a trace of anger or frustration.

We began Smokey on insulin injections, and he did well for a couple of months. Then, one day, Carol rushed him in. She had arrived home and found him having a seizure. Blood tests revealed he was hypoglycemic; his blood sugar was dangerously low. It was possible that both Carol and her son had given him his insulin. Some cats are hard to regulate, but a complication that severe was highly unusual, even with a double dose of insulin. We treated Smokey with intravenous dextrose, but he continued to seize off and on. It was nearly closing time at the clinic, and my patient was nowhere near stable. The clinic was not staffed overnight, and Carol could not afford to bring him to Tufts for continued overnight care. I didn't know what to do. Then, the clinic owner, Bart, suggested something I hadn't thought of.

"You could bring him home with you," he said.

I'd been in practice for three years, and it had never occurred to me to bring a patient home. Wait, that's not quite true. I'd brought home that one stray kitten with distemper in my first few months of practice, and it had died overnight. Waking up to find a dead kitten was something I'd tried to forget. And it meant I didn't exactly have a great track record. But Bart's idea made sense.

"All you can do," Bart continued, "is keep giving him valium through his IV catheter when he has a seizure." We knew the continued seizures were bad for Smokey's brain. We didn't know whether he would recover, but by bringing him home I could give him a chance. It was not something to offer to just any client, but I felt comfortable with Carol, who was relieved and grateful.

That night, I kept my own animals out of my bedroom and Smokey confined to a cat carrier next to my bed. He was sleepy from all the valium he'd already had. Every time my patient started thumping around in the carrier, I'd wake up and administer more valium very slowly through his IV, just enough so he stopped seizing. I worried about what all that medication was doing to him, but it was better than the seizures.

The next day, I brought Smokey back into work. To my great relief, his seizures had stopped. But he was groggy, and all he did was sleep. We kept him in the hospital to monitor his blood sugar, and Carol brought in something special to hang on his cage for good luck, a little cream-colored fleece teddy bear with golden wings, clasping a red rose in its paws. It must have been a Christmas ornament, as it had a string with a loop attached. Carol called it Smokey's "angel bear," and it made me smile every time I walked past his cage in the treatment area.

After a few days, Smokey's blood sugar was stable enough for him to go home. However, he was not the same cat. He had suffered permanent brain damage from his excessive seizures and seemed somewhat slow. Carol was happy to have him despite his change in personality, and we celebrated his release from the hospital. Maybe he would get back to his old self at home.

Unfortunately, Smokey didn't improve much. This wouldn't have been a problem except that he couldn't seem to remember to use the litter box. Smokey just urinated and defecated wherever he was. Carol tried to care for him as best she could, but after a few months, she called me.

"I try to bathe him, but he hates it, and he's just covered in poop all the time. He drags his tail in it and won't keep a diaper on," she explained. "My apartment is small, and I don't have room to keep him separated from the other cats. I don't think he'd like that anyways. He doesn't have a good quality of life anymore."

We had been through this already and tried a couple of different things. I knew this was a hard phone call for Carol to make.

"You've done so much for him," I said. "You know him better than anyone. If you don't think he has a good quality of life, it sounds like it's time."

Carol scheduled an appointment, and a few days later she, her son, Smokey, and I gathered in one of the exam rooms for the euthanasia. Smokey died peacefully, surrounded by family and me, the doctor who had tried to help him. After the injection, I felt the yearning I often had, of wanting the exact right words to appear, so I could say something helpful at this most difficult of times. On that day, words came to me.

"You know," I said, patting his soft fur, "Smokey may not have had his health, but he sure was loved." We cried and hugged.

As she left, Carol pressed something soft into my hands. I looked down to see Smokey's angel bear. "I want you to have it," she said. This time, I had no words.

Smokey's angel bear has hung in my home office ever since, reminding me of the love and commitment possible between animal and human.

Soon after Smokey died, I heard about a weeklong volunteer spay-neuter trip to the Dominican Republic sponsored by the state veterinary association. I was happy with my decision to remain in the United States, but I missed traveling. Dearly. I really wanted to go on the trip. But as a recent graduate who had just started her own business, I couldn't afford it, so I quickly dismissed the idea.

Shortly afterward, I received a phone call from the trip leader: an older veterinarian who couldn't make the trip had donated money to support another doctor's travel. Would I be interested? I was thrilled; the money would pay for about a quarter of the trip. Someone at work suggested that I ask the veterinary supply companies I had set up accounts with for donations, and the representatives agreed to donate some money. With half the trip paid for, I was able to fund the rest myself.

I was both the youngest veterinarian on the trip and the only woman out of seven doctors. Fortunately, this was not a disadvantage. The other doctors were glad I was there, and I did surgery with everyone else. Several of the doctors had brought their families, who acted as veterinary assistants. We worked hard, and ate dinners all together at a large table, sharing food and stories.

One day I noticed one of the doctors, Rich, working on a stray dog that had already had surgery and was still under anesthesia. Curious, I went over to ask what he was doing.

"Acupuncture!" he responded. I was surprised. I knew little about acupuncture, but I thought it was a very crunchy-granola treatment that didn't seem like this veterinarian at all. Rich had short gray hair and a no-nonsense manner. If anything, he looked like he would have thrived in the military.

Rich explained that acupuncture used tiny filament needles to access energy points in the dog's body. I could see for myself how thin the needles were. The dog he was treating had an old leg injury, and while he knew that one treatment wouldn't cure the problem, it would at least provide the dog with some pain relief. I was fascinated. I thought of Smokey, who had suffered serious complications from his medications. Perhaps if I'd had access to additional medical tools like holistic medicine, I could have helped him more. I stayed during the procedure and watched, not knowing how acupuncture would eventually change my life.

Five years later, Smokey and other pets like him finally inspired me to learn veterinary acupuncture. By then, I knew a few veterinarians who were utilizing acupuncture at their practices, including my friend Karen, who still lived and practiced in Maine. My colleagues enjoyed using acupuncture in conjunction with conventional Western medicine and were happy with the results they obtained. Acupuncture seemed intriguing and I found myself drawn to it. While I was not unhappy with my work, I was ready to try something new.

Unlike human medicine, where acupuncture is practiced mainly by licensed acupuncturists who are not Western-trained physicians, acupuncture on animals is performed by Western-trained, licensed veterinarians who have received additional training in veterinary acupuncture.

I realized I would need to travel out of state for training, as the nearest location for the course was in Florida. The schedule consisted of on-site lectures and training one week per month for four months, followed by a certification exam a month or two later. The full course would necessitate a total of five separate trips and over twenty nights of hotel stays. The cost of the program itself was several thousand dollars, and I'd have to contend with four weeks of lost income. As I was self-employed, I was not compensated for any of this by my employer. This was an expensive proposition, and I sadly realized I could not afford it. My dream of learning acupuncture would have to wait.

About a month later, I received a pamphlet in the mail. For the first time, the School of Veterinary Medicine at Tufts was offering an acupuncture course! My alma mater was only five miles from my house. If I subtracted the costs of travel and lodging, the amount was within my reach. I signed up immediately.

One of the reasons I could (just barely) afford the course is that most of my clients bought their heartworm and flea and tick prevention medications from me instead of a catalog company. In my business, this was a rare source of easy income, and helped offset the fact that it was difficult to charge enough for my services and keep them affordable. My suppliers continually raised prices, and I did not practice in a wealthy area. Charging enough was a constant struggle for me. Fortunately, many of my clients felt strongly about supporting small business owners, knowing their money was more likely to stay in their community if they "shopped local." Lately it's become more common for people to order their pet's prescriptions from online retailers, forcing doctors and staff to spend uncompensated time each day approving medications, writing scrips, and sending faxes and emails. If more people bought their supplies in their community, their clinic might be able to hire another receptionist to decrease telephone hold times, give their staff a much-needed raise, purchase costly life-saving equipment, or send a doctor to an expensive course such as acupuncture training.

After the course began, I realized how little I knew about acupuncture. I had known it would be another way to *treat* my patients, but I hadn't understood that it was also another way to *diagnose* them—an entirely different system of medicine called Traditional Chinese Medicine, or TCM. I also hadn't realized how hard it would be to learn something new and different; I needed to have much of the information repeated many times before it sunk in. However, I was fascinated. I learned new parts to the physical exam I had performed so many times on so many animals—looking at the animal's tongue and taking the pulse. I thought about Oupa; his first step if I wasn't feeling well was always to take my pulse. I wished he were still alive so I could discuss pulse-taking with him.

One aspect of learning acupuncture involved memorizing the acupuncture point locations, which were all anatomical. I unearthed one of my old veterinary school textbooks, rarely used in my current practice, titled *Anatomy of the Dog*. Rana was a willing model. With her short coat, it was easy to find the acupuncture point locations I needed to learn. Trudy was older and grumpy, and she had been there for me as I went through veterinary school, when I used to seek her out to feel her lymph nodes or whatever else we were studying (being the pet of a veterinary student had its drawbacks). She had paid her dues, so I let her be.

As I continued with the course, things that had never made sense before began to fall into place. I learned that Traditional Chinese Veterinary Medicine, or TCVM, regards the patient with a wide-angle view that includes all body systems, the patient's environment, and even the animal's temperament. The patient is seen as an individual rather than as representative of a disease. Instead of identifying separate problems, TCVM paints all the animal's issues into one big picture and looks for patterns. Suddenly, it meant something that a dog might have both chronic ear infections and anal gland problems. While Western medicine may not connect the two issues, TCVM sees them as two symptoms of the same underlying problem, affecting areas on the same meridian or energy channels. It was a good fit for the way I practiced, as my house calls had led me to try to understand my patients' life stories.

TCVM, I found, was a great complement to Western veterinary medicine, as it excelled at treating the very issues I struggled to treat in my patients: chronic problems. It was often beneficial to utilize both systems of medicine in the same patient, which is called integrative medicine, integrating Western and holistic medicine to achieve the best of both worlds. An animal might benefit from a certain medication, but by utilizing acupuncture, I might be able to decrease or eliminate the pet's dosage and thus the risk of side effects.

TCVM is a complex system of medicine, much of which has been extrapolated from human TCM. One part is termed Five Elements, or Five Phases, which includes a way of looking at different personality types, also called constitutions. While everyone likely has some elements of each personality type, and certain ones tend to be more prominent at different stages of one's life and in different seasons, there is often one type of constitution that stands out. Certain constitutions are prone to certain problems. Now I saw patterns in my patients that I had been unaware of, and it felt as though a light had been turned on. This was more than another tool in the toolbox; it was like finding a whole new toolshed.

It was fascinating to look at animals and people with this new lens. I considered Rana to have a Fire constitution, due to her high energy level, joyful nature, and love of socializing. Trudy, who loved to be in charge, was a Wood element. Mike, who favored routine and logic, had a Metal constitution (as one teacher noted, "We want our air traffic controllers to have a Metal constitution"). My cat, Daiquiri, with his sweet disposition, calm and agreeable nature, and low energy level fit the description of an Earth constitution. I myself, I concluded, was somewhere between an Earth (especially due to my tendency to worry) and a Fire. These terms became a part of my vocabulary, and Mike's, too; we would sometimes describe a person as being "very Metal" or "a real Fire personality."

Part of the study of TCVM involved learning to think in metaphors. A commonly used metaphor is the yin-yang symbol, the circle with the swirl and the two dots.

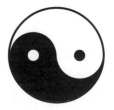

One side is light, and the other dark, with the dots having the inverse colors. In our society, we tend to think in terms of opposites and absolutes: black and white, good and evil, right and wrong. The yin-yang symbol represents yin and yang as being opposites, yet both are equally valuable and important. The symbol demonstrates that there is no day without night, no light without darkness, no activity without calm. Anyone who has ever suffered from insomnia would agree that there is no wake without sleep. No matter which way the yin-yang circle is bisected, the result will contain some of both yin and yang, of light and dark. This further emphasizes the equality of both halves.

In our culture, we tend to disparage darkness, using the word to represent something undesirable, which has always bothered me. Why do we say "dark thoughts" when we mean unhappy or unpleasant thoughts? I wondered if this tendency was rooted in racism. In any case, the trend is so pervasive that even black dogs and cats are the last to be adopted in our animal shelters, a phenomenon termed "black dog syndrome" or "black dog bias."

I didn't realize how involved I had become in my new study, and how excited about acupuncture and TCVM I was, until Mike commented one day, "What did we used to talk about before you started learning acupuncture?"

The following year, Tufts offered the acupuncture course again. Although I had already taken and passed the two-day exam, completed my internship hours and case report, and obtained my veterinary acupuncture certification, I decided to become a teaching assistant for the course. That way, I could attend any lectures I wanted to for free. I wanted to hear some of the information again, to explore some of the concepts more fully. I also enjoy teaching, and it was fun to introduce other veterinarians to acupuncture.

Rana became my point model for the anatomy labs we held to show students the point locations. The first time she came with me to the lab, she had fun greeting all the other veterinarians until she noticed a dog skeleton mounted on a table. Suddenly, every hackle on her body stood up as she crouched in obvious canine confusion and fear. I don't know if the model was a real skeleton or not, but she clearly recognized the smell or the shape of the model, which we quickly hid. With the dog skeleton out of sight, Rana loved coming to Tufts and being patted and spoiled as I taught. She thus was able to help many veterinarians learn acupuncture.

One Sunday morning, not long after I finished acupuncture training, we were all (humans and animals) hanging out on our enclosed back porch with a view of the lake. Mike and I were reading the Sunday newspaper and sipping our tea when there was a sudden loud commotion—Daiquiri, my sweet and now elderly cat, was attacking Rana fiercely, with claws, teeth, and primal yowls. We separated them and tried to piece together what had happened. Rana had been lying peacefully on the floor in the sun, and Daiquiri had gone over to her. I knew then that something was very wrong with my gentle cat.

In hindsight, Daiquiri had not been himself for some time before this incident. He had been restless and acting strange. The more I thought about it, the more I was convinced he had been having headaches.

Most people don't think of animals as being affected by headaches. However, it's likely many species suffer from headaches, just as people do. Dogs and cats seldom vocalize with a chronic type of pain or an ache. Instead, they will simply sleep more, isolate themselves, and perhaps not act 100 percent themselves. When Mike and I discussed Daiquiri's behavior, we also identified a few times we had seen him head-pressing, or pushing his head firmly against something—the sofa, me, Rana. This is something animals may do as an attempt to relieve the pain of a headache. It was a new behavior for Dai, and it strengthened my belief that his head was hurting him. We concluded that Dai had head-pressed against Rana right before he attacked her.

I ran some routine blood work on Daiquiri, which was normal. Next, I scheduled an abdominal ultrasound for him, which was also normal. I was slowly eliminating things that could be wrong with my friend. Eventually, I scheduled an appointment for Daiquiri with a veterinary neurologist at Tufts. At the hospital, the neurologist reviewed my cat's behavior and test results and performed a full neurological exam. Finally, he told me that yes, my cat might well have a brain tumor. The only way to find out would be to perform an MRI of his head.

I wrestled with my decision. On the one hand, he was a fifteen-year-old cat who had lived a long and happy life. No one would fault me for not going forward with an expensive procedure that was, after all, purely diagnostic and would do nothing to treat Daiquiri's underlying problem, whatever it was. In fact, one could argue it would be foolish to proceed, and several family members and friends did so.

On the other hand, deep inside me, I felt a pull, a feeling I could not ignore. I needed to *know*.

This need for information was something I had seen before. Certainly, a part of my desire to know what was wrong with Dai came from my medical background; doctors tend to prefer certainty, and we are trained to find answers to questions, to figure out *why*. I had also seen many clients request information even when faced with an animal gravely sick or injured, to gain the peace of mind to make a euthanasia decision with a clear conscience and to ensure a diagnosis was correct. Sometimes veterinarians have conclusive information to give to clients about their pet's condition, and sometimes we don't. It is always easier when a client can look at an X-ray or blood test results and understand why their animal is in distress. If Dai did not have a brain tumor, I reasoned, perhaps there was something else going on, something that could be treated. Admittedly, however, a part of my decision was based not on logic but on a strong feeling of intuition.

Daiquiri had his MRI, which identified two small tumors on his brain. The neurologist explained that, at the time, there was a limited database of MRIs of feline brains, which made it harder to interpret. Exactly how the masses were causing his symptoms was unclear. In terms of treatment, he said, surgery would be difficult, but radiation was a possibility. I shook my head. Dai had been incredibly stressed by leaving the house and visiting the hospital, so bringing him back multiple times was out of the question unless it would dramatically improve the outcome. I concluded I was likely going to have to euthanize my precious cat, although at least now I knew why. Yet Daiquiri was my first cat, and the thought of letting him go was devastating.

Dai's MRI took place during the week I was attending an herbal medicine TCVM seminar at Tufts given by my favorite teacher from the veterinary acupuncture course, a Canadian veterinarian named Steve Marsden. I decided to ask Steve if he would examine Daiquiri. It was a big ask, and I was nervous; Steve was a rock star in the holistic veterinary world, and long lines of doctors waited to ask him questions during the breaks between lectures.

At the next break, I asked Steve if he would examine my own cat, and whether I could pay him for the consult. Steve proposed a visit to my house after class the following day to look at Dai and see him in his own environment. I was amazed and grateful.

Eileen was the veterinarian who owned the clinic where I worked part-time, and she had become a mentor. She also did acupuncture, and I invited her to come over for Steve's consult. We watched as Steve gently examined Daiquiri in my home. He asked many questions about Dai and his habits and personality, such as if he liked to lie in the sun, and whether he was friendly or shy—questions that made no diagnostic sense in Western veterinary medicine terms. Steve focused intently as he performed an advanced technique, placing an acupuncture needle in my cat's leg and then checking to see if Dai's pulse had changed. Finally he turned to us. He explained that in TCVM, Daiquiri was suffering from excessive dampness, a common diagnosis in Chinese medicine. *Dampness* meant he was not adequately processing his food, and the byproducts were accumulating in his body and becoming toxic. Steve recommended a dietary change and prescribed some Chinese herbs. When I asked what I owed him, Steve just shrugged, and I wrote a check for what I could afford.

I had nothing to lose. I switched Dai's food and gave him the herbs. To Mike's and my amazement, within three weeks Daiquiri was back to normal, with no evidence of his prior agitation or discomfort. No more head-pressing or restlessness. No more cranky kitty. He was his old sweet, happy, gentle self. Even Steve seemed surprised his recommendations had worked so well—he was back in Canada, but I kept him updated via email. I would have loved to repeat the MRI, to see if the tumors had changed, but the expense was prohibitive. I continued the herbs and the new food, and from that time forward, enjoyed every day with my cat as a bonus day.

Daiquiri's symptoms never returned. I was so grateful that I'd had access to those ideas, which were outside the mainstream veterinary practice in the United States. I knew I would never ignore my new tool kit again.

When I went to California to visit my college friend Robin a few months later, Mike took care of Trudy, Rana, and Daiquiri. Shortly after I returned, we went out for a nice dinner. When we got home, Mike proposed, offering me a ring he'd carved out of a giant Hershey bar while I was away. He knew that chocolate was far more important to me than diamonds. I knew my answer was yes.

9

Dog of Honor

One of my acupuncture house-call patients was a geriatric golden retriever, Leah, who had been struggling to go up the few stairs into her house. I arrived one day to find a newly built ramp blocking the front steps. "I was going to have it by the kitchen door," the dog's owner explained, "but it wouldn't fit. So, I thought, who needs a front door anyway?" Clearly, Leah's comfort took priority over the access to her own front door. I loved this about her.

While pets are not our children, there are some similarities in the relationships. We are responsible for our animals, for their food, shelter, and well-being. We raise them, teach them, clean up after them (oh, how we clean up after them!). They depend on us, yet we can depend on them in ways we should not depend on our children—for continued companionship and unconditional love. We are not raising our pets to leave the nest, to be independent. Our expectations for them are different from what they are for our children, and thus our relationships are less complicated; more like friendship, perhaps, than a parent-child relationship.

Lately it seems as though we don't even know what to call them. When I was in veterinary school, the human half of the human-animal unit was always referred to as the owner. Recently, letters from a local veterinary referral center have changed their description from *owner* to *guardian*. For animals, the term *fur baby* is currently favored by many, although others strongly dislike it. While working with dogs or cats, veterinarians (myself included) and technicians will often talk to the pet: *It's okay, Olive, just look at Mom, we'll be done in a minute* or *Don't worry, honey, Dad's right there.*

Stella was a little cat who lived with an elderly woman named Dora in senior low-income housing. The front door of the apartment opened into a small dining area, where I sat down at the table to talk to Stella's owner before examining her.

I couldn't help observing that most of the walls of the living and dining areas were covered with pictures from magazines, calendars, and postcards. The decor appeared to have two general themes: cats and Christianity, each receiving approximately equal consideration. Everywhere I looked were photos of cats and kittens, as well as crosses and religious quotes.

Eventually we discussed Stella's diet. I could see her food bowls in the galley kitchen, and I got up to have a closer look—one of the advantages of house-call practice. I remarked about the adorable springtime-themed vinyl place mat upon which Stella's food and water bowls rested.

"Oh yes," replied Dora, obviously pleased. "I swap them out seasonally. I have several different place mats for her."

Dora's sister was there for the appointment, and I presumed they lived together. "Can you *believe* how spoiled that cat is?" she asked, feigning an eye roll. "How many cats get *seasonal place mats?*"

We all had a good laugh about Stella and her special place mats, and I felt warmed by Dora's affection for her beloved cat. Of course, Stella herself was unaware of the place mats, which were likely purchased at the local dollar store.

Every so often, I come across a newspaper or magazine story about how we spoil our pets to excess. The writer will list such things as flavored water for pets, designer collars and clothing, and complex medical care as proof that we have lost our collective minds when it comes to how we treat our animals.

Many of my clients spend a lot of money on their pets' care, not because they are wealthy, but because their animals are a high priority for them. However, the act of spending money on a pet's care is far more likely to be judged harshly in comparison with the same amount going toward a new car, the latest electronics, a kitchen remodel, or trips to a casino. If the price tag for an animal's medical care heads up into the thousands, there may be people who believe the money should instead be donated to a children's charity. Somehow, the act of spending money on a beloved pet risks being judged as evidence of a broad rejection of humanity in favor of the animal kingdom.

A colleague once referred an acupuncture case to me for a house call. Afterward, she said, "I just have to ask. Those clients have spent thousands and thousands on their animals at Tufts. What was their house like?"

"You know," I replied, "it was a pretty ordinary small ranch house. Nothing special."

This was quite common. Clients who lived in large or fancy houses were no more likely to spend money on, say, blood work or specialists for their animals than people who lived in more modest homes or apartments. The care people took of their animals depended on their pet's value to them, not where they lived or how much money they had.

———

Much of the time, the spoiling of our animals is something we do for ourselves, and doing home visits allowed me to see all kinds of whimsical things created for animal family members. At Christmastime, the area above my patient Cesar's cat door sported a holiday wreath with a large red bow. Another feline patient had family photos taped to the inside of the cabinet where his cat food was stored, to create the look of a school locker. At Dick and Claire's house, pig paraphernalia was everywhere, including a framed jigsaw puzzle featuring flying pigs. Arnell also had a giant litter box in the bedroom so she could sleep in the same room with them. Our animals' lives are intertwined with our own, physically, emotionally, even spiritually—as they should be, because, unless something goes wrong, ours is the only home they'll ever know. We thus have a responsibility to them that is different from our responsibility to our children, yet no less sacred.

Medical care aside, we don't need to spend a lot of money to spoil our pets; the best-loved pets are spoiled with attention and love. Animals have an amazing ability to be who they are, in all their otherness, and at the same time to offer companionship and love to humans, adjusting to our lives in their own unique ways. They don't care whether they are called "fur baby" or not. Our pets don't just give us unconditional love, they accept our love unconditionally, in whichever way we choose to give it.

"Since my kids moved out, I have her lick the spoon when I'm finished cooking," one client confessed. Holly the Australian shepherd was definitely the dog of the household, yet she didn't mind rising to the occasion and licking an occasional spoon.

Most cat owners realize the likelihood of a cat appreciating a toy or other item bought for their entertainment is inversely proportional to the amount of money spent on said item. Cats are notoriously hard to buy for, and many would rather play with the plastic ring from a milk container or hop inside an empty cardboard box than bother with some expensive toy. Yet we still get toys for them. We love them. And sometimes they are thrilled with the catnip mouse or cat tree or crinkly cat mat we picked out just for them, and we feel as though we have won the lottery.

People sometimes ask me whether we spoil our animals too much. This has always seemed an odd question to me, like asking whether we love our animals too much. The only way we can spoil them "too much" is by overfeeding them. Obesity is a health crisis among pets as well as people, and I have heard all manner of *food is love* excuses. I once had the following conversation with a client.

Me. Well, I have to tell you, Bailey is obese. We've checked his thyroid, and the level is normal. So we need to focus on changing your dog's diet, and hopefully you can also get him to exercise more. At this weight, he's at higher risk for diabetes and heart disease as well as arthritis. Can you tell me what you are feeding him now?

Client. You know, it's hard to believe, but he only gets a cup of food twice a day, and that's it.

Me. Any table food?

Client. Nope, none at all. We're very particular about that.

Me. Okay, what about cookies then?

Client. Oh, he has as many of those as he wants.

Me, *frowning in confusion.* As many as he wants?

Client, *with a shrug.* Sure, he knows where they're kept, and he can open the cupboard door. If he wants a cookie, he goes and gets one.

In our culture, the prevalent assumption is that animals are entirely inferior to humans. Yet, although most animals don't have opposable thumbs or our type of cognitive abilities, they undoubtedly have many skills we don't possess, and we may have only begun to tap the surface of their capabilities.

Imagine the information dogs obtain from their sense of smell, estimated to be ten thousand to one hundred thousand times as sensitive as that of a human; in the future, we may use dog noses to routinely screen for common diseases. Dogs work in airport security and drug detection, help autistic children to communicate, act as comfort animals after tragedies, and perform numerous other important jobs.

How does your cat know when you are upset? How does your dog know you are about to come home? These species have lived with humans, side by side, for thousands of years; they may know us better than we know ourselves.

Non-animal-lovers sometimes question whether animal people are guilty of anthropomorphizing. Recently, studies have demonstrated that dogs can experience a wide range of emotions, something that is unsurprising to most dog lovers. Personally, I have witnessed dogs and cats I believe are experiencing the emotions of joy, sadness, contentment, disdain (cats really shine here), anger, longing, jealousy, and anxiety, among other feelings.

When I recognize an emotion in an animal, wild or domesticated, I get the same feeling as when I recognize the commonality in someone from another culture, another country, who experiences a different way of life. The wonderful aha moment of *Yes! Really? Me too!* It is one of the reasons I love to travel. The differences may be fantastic—different food, cities, vistas, ways of life, languages—but it is the finding of similarities within the differences that never fails to amaze me.

One of the ways I enjoy experiencing this sharing of "humanity" in the animal kingdom is simply watching an animal yawn and stretch. Yes, each species has its own way of stretching; cats may spread their toes, some dogs lift their tails at the end. But the stretching and what it feels like to stretch—these are the same. When we perform a cat pose or downward dog pose in yoga, we are imitating these stretches.

And we know our animals love us, despite those who doubt that nonhumans are capable of love. After all, how can one measure love? Can emotion possibly be corralled into double-blind controlled studies and quantified? While oxytocin has been called the love hormone and can be measured in humans and animals, emotions such as love may be better understood through art, such as songs and poems, rather than scientific research. Anyone who has ever shared the affection of an animal can only feel bad for those who have never experienced such a connection.

Our misunderstandings about animals often result from failing to take their differences into account. The behaviors that send dogs and cats to animal shelters are usually normal actions for the species, yet they are behaviors we humans view as incompatible with our own lifestyles. A dog who chews up a leather shoe is exhibiting normal dog behavior, as is a cat who refuses to use a tiny enclosed litter box that hasn't been cleaned in a week. It is up to us to meet them at least halfway, by figuring out their needs and providing for them—more chew toys and exercise for the dog (as well as limited access to shoes), and a clean uncovered litter box for the cat.

Some genuine anthropomorphizing is done purely for human amusement, such as when we pretend animals are speaking our language, as seen in many animal videos on social media as well as in television, movies, and cartoons. Although I used to cringe when I saw these types of videos, I do enjoy some of them. I usually consider them harmless, provided we remember that we are envisioning what a human would say under those circumstances and that animals don't exist merely for our entertainment. On the plus side, when we wonder how an animal might feel, and how it compares to how we ourselves would feel in a situation, it may help us relate to animals better. It is also beneficial for our imagination and sense of play, which for many of us get far too little use.

There is one common type of anthropomorphizing that can be harmful. Veterinary behaviorists' research has demonstrated dogs and cats do not experience guilt or shame. This makes sense, given their ability to live in the moment.

What are we observing, then, in the numerous "dog shaming" video clips, in which dogs are confronted with evidence of their misdeeds and respond with flattened ears, downcast facial expressions, and averted eyes?

We are witnessing canine anxiety. Dogs can tell from a person's tone of voice and body language that they are angry. They would react the same whether they had done something to incur the anger or not. Dogs and cats also do not act out of a desire to seek revenge or to get back at their owners. An animal that makes a mess— say, defecating on the floor—is either exhibiting normal behavior (the litter box is full), has a medical condition, or is stressed and anxious. When viewed with this lens, those videos meant to seem amusing instead appear cruel. I hope that as more people realize this, the shaming photos and videos will end.

I wonder whether their very inability to experience shame and remorse draws us to animals. Those emotions may drive human behavior more than we realize. Dr. Brené Brown, a writer and researcher studying shame and vulnerability, has referred to shame as an "unspoken epidemic." Perhaps it's a relief to be in the company of creatures who are seemingly immune to these emotions, in both themselves and others. While someone may experience embarrassment in front of their spouse, child, parent, coworker, boss, neighbor, or friend, it is nearly impossible to be embarrassed in front of one's pet. Animals don't judge—who else would you feel comfortable having in the bathroom with you? They don't care what we look like or how we dress; they know us by our smell. With our pets, we are shielded from shame and guilt; we can reveal the broken places we all have inside us, knowing they will never laugh or poke fun. Our secrets are safe with them.

These days, when much of our communication is virtual, it is not only refreshing but vital to interact with a real, live creature. We touch, and are touched by, our pets. They ground us in both time and place. Our pets *see* us—really see us, and we see them. They welcome us when we arrive home, and we smile, despite the long day. We feel their weight, on our laps, on our beds.

Animals also have an uncanny ability to bring humans together, helping us understand one another and build bridges. If we can agree about animals, perhaps we can agree—or agree to disagree—about other things.

One November, Mike and I happened to be visiting my father and Angela at their condo in Florida during a presidential election due to a family wedding. I was excited for the opportunity to hold signs for the candidate I supported while in a swing state, and we bought some poster boards and made signs—mine said VETERINARIANS FOR KERRY. On the day of the election, Mike and I headed down the street to the local polling place, along with Petey the spaniel.

Election Day in Florida turned out to be quite different than in Massachusetts, at least as far as the weather was concerned. Instead of bundling up in sweaters and coats, we wore shorts and T-shirts, and carried plenty of water for ourselves and the dog. We chose a spot the requisite number of feet away near some other Kerry supporters, and settled down in some lawn chairs under an umbrella. We chatted with voters, and Petey received plenty of attention from us and from people walking by.

We spotted the Bush contingency a short distance away. One woman in particular stood out. She was smartly dressed in red, white, and blue from head to toe, including a bandstand-style hat.

Her clothes were festooned with patriotic ribbons, and she carried a large American flag in addition to her sizable BUSH sign. Her makeup was flawless. Despite the warm weather, she paraded back and forth for hours.

At one point, the woman appeared to be heading in our direction. I clutched Mike's arm, having no idea what to make of her approach. Would she yell at us? Did she know we were from out of state? Suddenly, I felt distinctly underdressed in my casual attire.

As I had feared, the woman made eye contact as she got closer. I braced myself as her Southern-accented voice rang out.

"That *dog* is *precious!*"

There, outside a swing state's polling place during a heavily contested presidential election, two Democrats and a Republican stood in complete agreement over a dog.

"You can't have a dog in a wedding!" said Mike.

"Why not, though?" I asked. "We're going to have it outside anyways. I wouldn't trust her in the house."

We had rented a historical home in a nearby town and hoped to hold the ceremony outdoors if the weather permitted.

"But who would hold on to her?" Mike asked.

"Lisa or Karen," I responded eagerly. Then I frowned. "I wouldn't have her at the reception, though. She'd be on top of tables with her face in the food." I brightened as I thought of a solution: "Someone could bring her back to my dad and Angela's house; it's so close to the wedding."

Mike still looked skeptical.

"Rana's so friendly, she would have a great time. Trudy, on the other hand, would just be stressed. And I'm sure the minister won't mind," I added. We had hired a Unitarian Universalist minister I'd met a few years earlier because she had adopted a dog I'd rescued.

The dog had been brought into the clinic by the local shelter for me to euthanize, but he had tried to lick me through his muzzle. Instead of euthanizing him, I brought him home overnight, and then to the Buddy Dog shelter the following day, where he had been adopted by the minister within a week.

We had also hired a local musician who had been one of my clients before she moved closer to Boston. The wedding was full of dog people.

"Would she have to do something, like carry the rings?" Mike looked doubtful.

"Oh God, no," I responded with a shudder. "She'd lose them in a minute. No, she doesn't have to *do* anything except be there. She can be the Dog of Honor."

"Hmm ... Interspecies representative?"

"Yes! I love it!"

Mike shook his head and sighed. "Well, you are a veterinarian ..."

About a week before the wedding, weather forecasters warned about a large hurricane on a path to travel up the coast. I worried; although we had the option of holding the ceremony indoors, we also had family members and friends flying in from across the country. What if people couldn't come?

That day, I did a house call for a dalmatian named Joe. Veterinarians know that the breed, which increased in popularity after the 101 *Dalmatians* movies, are not always the family-friendly dogs portrayed in the films; they can be timid and unpredictable. Joe, however, was a sweet, friendly dog who loved everyone. Joe's owner, Liz, knew I was getting married, and we discussed the impending storm.

"This happened to one of my relatives with her wedding," Liz recalled.

"Really? What happened?" I asked.

"She tried this old-wives'-tale trick of hanging a string of rosary beads out her bedroom window before the wedding, and it
worked!"

"No kidding," I responded.

"Her wedding day was fine! I think I have a rosary if you want
to try it," said Liz.

I took the rosary beads home and told Mike. A weather junkie,
he had been following the predicted path of the storm, and it didn't
look good. "Hey, whatever," he said, and we headed up the stairs to
put the rosary beads outside our bedroom window.

A couple of days later, the forecast showed a completely different path for the storm. Rather than follow along the coast, it was
instead heading far inland and would completely bypass eastern
Massachusetts.

"This is a very unusual path; I've never seen a storm do this before," remarked the weather forecaster. Mike and I looked at each
other wide-eyed.

Liz was thrilled, too, and I was glad she'd been involved in an
aspect of my wedding, however small. I'd felt like extended family
for many of my clients, and it was nice to feel that they could act as
my extended family as well.

My friends wove flowers into Rana's collar. Mike smiled and relaxed
as he watched Rana walk up the aisle with Lisa (we later learned
that one of Mike's aunts mistook her for a guide dog). I took my
place under the chuppah we had fashioned out of a vintage embroidered tablecloth belonging to my grandmother. Then in her nine-
ties, she'd been unable to make the long flight from South Africa
for the wedding. The sun shone through the embroidered openings
in the cloth, creating beautiful patterns on the grass underneath.

As I joined Mike in front of the minister, I became aware of a
familiar noise behind me.

It was Rana, panting.

Perhaps she was thirsty, or maybe she was wondering why everyone was standing and sitting so quietly and why she couldn't continue to run around greeting people. Perhaps she was excited because everyone she loved was there. Maybe she wanted to get closer to me. Whatever the reason, Rana's breath behind us was a grounding presence for both Mike and me throughout the ceremony, as we transitioned from single to married.

She was not just a part of our lives. She was family.

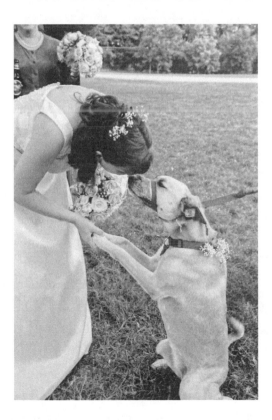

10

The Universe Shifts

I can pinpoint the exact moment everything changed.

I was sitting at the kitchen table with Rana sprawled beside me on the floor. I was probably reading the newspaper or looking out at the lake. In my mind, that is labeled "Before."

And then, for no reason I can think of, no reason at all, I reached down and lifted my dog's upper lip, revealing the teeth and the gums below. There, above her right upper canine tooth, the gum looked funny.

"Huh," I said out loud.

Everything else was "After."

I got down onto the floor to have a better look. The area did look strange. It wasn't very big, only about the size of a dime, but I didn't know if I had ever seen anything quite like it before. The gum area was enlarged and thickened. I checked the left side of Rana's mouth. That side looked normal.

I didn't know what to make of it. It didn't look like a big deal . . . but I had a funny feeling.

If I had seen something similar on one of my patients, I know what I would have done. I would have said to the dog's owner, "I don't know what it is. It does look strange, but it's not very big. It's not bothering her, so that's good. Maybe the area is temporarily inflamed for some reason. Let's try a course of antibiotics. Come back in two weeks, and we'll have another look. If nothing has changed, we may want to consider a biopsy."

That was not what I did. I called the veterinary dental specialist in my area and made an appointment. Although we could have done a biopsy at the clinic I worked at, I listened to my intuition and went straight to the specialist.

A week or so later, at the veterinary dentist's office, Rana charmed the staff. There was an unusual table in the exam room, with built-in stairs for the patient to climb. Rana happily climbed right up onto the exam table as I remarked that I had never seen one like it, and Dr. Laura LeVan, the veterinary dentist, explained that it was custom-made. I was nervous, so I made small talk.

Finally I showed her the area in Rana's mouth. In that room, consulting with a specialist, a colleague, I managed to find words for the fear that had been troubling me since I first noticed the area.

"You know, it almost looks like it could be, uh, cancer . . . except she's only four years old," I said quietly, meaning, *So you and I both know that's not possible.* At the time, I had never seen cancer in a dog so young.

Laura, who was very pleasant, did not meet my eye, and I did not press her for a response. She concluded her exam, then recommended putting Rana under anesthesia so she could take a closer look, as well as dental X-rays and possibly a biopsy. I scheduled Rana for the next available appointment.

The day of Rana's procedure ended up being my half birthday, which I hoped was a good sign. However, due to heavy downpours, Rana and I ended up stuck in an awful highway traffic jam on the way to the dental office. Rana tended to be restless in the car, and with all the stop-and-go driving, it was an uncomfortable ride for both of us. We were more than a half hour late. I checked Rana into the dental clinic and arrived at my own clinic workplace shaken and distracted. A few hours later, the receptionist let me know I had a phone call.

I picked up the phone. Laura's voice was kind, but her words impaled me.

"It's cancer," she said right away. "I'm so sorry, Karen. I could tell as soon as I cut into it that it was a tumor and not normal gum tissue. We won't know what type of cancer it is until we get the biopsy report, but I'm guessing it's either squamous cell carcinoma or fibrosarcoma."

I started crying right away, even though I was at work. It had not occurred to me that we would know right away if it was cancer. I didn't know much about either kind of tumor, but I knew enough to know this was very bad news. My worst fears had been confirmed, and they swirled around me and condensed.

I told her I would do anything, anything at all to treat Rana.

"Look," Laura said, "let me set up an appointment with an oncologist at the Tufts small-animal hospital for you and Rana for as soon as possible. We'll have the biopsy results by the time of your appointment."

I agreed.

"Rana is *so* sweet," Laura added. "She is in everyone's lap as she is waking up from anesthesia. She's a lovely dog."

I nodded, tears running down my cheeks. "Yes, she is," I managed. "She's a great dog."

Everything that happened next seemed to blur together. Tears, phone calls, and an appointment at Tufts. Mike and I meeting with a veterinary oncologist. Although I can recall other important moments of Rana's diagnosis in painstaking detail, I have no memories of being in the exam room at Tufts that spring day; but I will never forget what we learned.

Rana's biopsy had shown a type of tumor called a fibrosarcoma. It was termed a maxillary fibrosarcoma due to its location on her maxilla, or upper jaw. It was a tumor that tended to grow locally and become invasive; it was an extremely aggressive type of cancer. However, the cells do not typically spread, or metastasize, to other parts of the body. Complete removal was the ideal treatment. If they could surgically remove the tumor, Rana might actually be cured. Cured! However, this would require a major surgery to remove part of her mouth and jaw. I couldn't imagine my precious dog with part of her face missing as the best possible scenario, but I accepted what the oncologist said. Cure would mean a normal life span.

The next step would be an MRI of Rana's head, so the oncologists and surgeons at Tufts could evaluate the extent of the tumor. The MRI would need to be done under anesthesia so she would stay completely still. If all looked okay, she would go immediately to surgery on the same day, while still under anesthesia.

Within two weeks of Rana's diagnosis, she was scheduled for the MRI and surgery. Waiting was hard—I kept imagining my dog after the surgery, with part of her face missing. Rana had no issues during this time, although the area where the biopsy had been taken seemed more swollen than before. Naturally, I checked it constantly, but Rana didn't seem to mind.

On the appointed day, I dropped Rana off at the Foster Hospital for Small Animals at Tufts, electing to wait at home rather than at the hospital. I knew working would be out of the question. Mike was at work, but Lisa, who had a flexible schedule, came over to help me wait. We sat around anxiously until the phone rang and I grabbed it. It was the surgeon, a woman I knew slightly; we had been in veterinary school at about the same time.

"We can't do the surgery," she said.

I felt the floor fall out from under me.

"The MRI showed that the tumor is already on the bottom of your dog's nasal cavity. We can do this surgery only if we believe we can remove all of the tumor, or she will go through this difficult surgery and recovery but the tumor will still come back," the surgeon explained.

As much as I didn't want Rana to have the surgery, I didn't want to hear this news. I was glad it came from someone I knew. I also felt my medical training surfacing; *Surgeons like to cut,* said a small voice inside my head, recalling a common phrase in medicine. *Surgery is what they do.* If a surgeon is telling me she can't do the surgery, I realized, I must believe her.

"You can come and see her," she continued. "She's waking up now. Just come on back to the anesthesia recovery ward."

Lisa and I jumped into the car. When we arrived at the recovery ward, Rana picked her head up and looked at me, bleary-eyed. Her tail wagged extra hard to see Lisa. I opened the door of the cage and sat down inside it, cradling her head in my lap. Lisa and I talked to Rana and patted her and told her what a wonderful dog she was.

Then we brought her home.

During my second year of practice, I surgically removed a cyst from Trudy's back, administering an intravenous anesthesia injection while a veterinary assistant held her. The procedure was uneventful, yet afterward I couldn't help thinking about how strange it had been to see her lying there on the surgery table, unconscious, hooked up to the anesthesia machine with an endotracheal tube sticking out of her mouth. The skin and tissue under the blue surgical drape looked like any other I had worked with, yet if I glanced away, I saw my own dog's brindled paws, so familiar and dear to me. Veterinarians typically pride themselves on their self-sufficiency, and most vets I knew treated their own animals. But the next time Trudy needed something, I mused, maybe I would ask a trusted colleague to do the surgery.

While I often take it in stride if my own animals are sick, I have noticed that sometimes, a strange thing happens: my doctor side recedes, and my pet owner side takes over. *Oh no! She's sick—what's wrong?* I might ask myself. *Why is Trudy vomiting?*

Okay, relax, my vet side will respond. Think about what you would ask a client. How about, could she have gotten into something that may have made her sick?

No, I don't think so, but maybe she had too many leftovers yesterday.

Okay, so that could be why. Is there any diarrhea, and is she acting okay?

No diarrhea, and she is acting fine. So what do I do?

What would I tell a client? Give her a bland diet for a few days and keep a close eye on her.

Okay, I can do that.

I think she'll be fine.

Phew.

Most of my pets' problems until that point had been relatively minor, except for Daiquiri's brain tumor. Even that, as stressful as it was, had occurred when he was an old cat. Rana was just entering the prime of her life. It had been only a few months since she had walked down the aisle in our wedding. I had never encountered something of this magnitude before, and I knew I would need support. In a sense, I was in the position of a layperson.

Even now, I recall the time surrounding Rana's diagnosis as one of the most difficult periods of my life. For years afterward, springtime—normally one of my favorite times of year—triggered an "anniversary reaction" of depression. My sensitivity to the difficulty of receiving a bad diagnosis spurred me to write an article for *The Bark* magazine entitled "How to Cope with a Serious Diagnosis: Ten Tips for Navigating Tough Decisions about Your Dog."[‡]

I thought about my client Gloria, and how she'd had to ask for help to care for her cats.

One morning, I picked up my business line to find Gloria's friendly voice on the other end. Gloria was an elderly woman who lived by herself and didn't have family in the area. She had two cats, whom she doted on and who kept her company. I expected her to say that something was wrong with one of her cats, but instead, she had called to ask if I knew of a pet-sitter who could feed them. I asked if she was going away, and she clarified that she was calling from the hospital; she had been admitted unexpectedly and was worried about her kitties.

Gloria lived in a small apartment in a poor neighborhood. She didn't have much money. In fact, she hadn't called me in a couple of years, I suspected, for this very reason. It was a holiday week, and I was sure the pet-sitters I knew were booked. "Don't worry," I said. "I'll make sure they're taken care of."

I asked Lisa to help me feed the cats as she lived closer to Gloria than I did. Lisa and her husband, Joe, were glad to help, so we split the care of the cats.

I called Gloria every day to let her know how her cats were doing and check in on her. Knowing she didn't have close friends or family nearby, I asked if she needed anything from home. Gloria asked me to bring her false teeth from the bathroom medicine cabinet. So I did.

Gloria was in the hospital for a week. When at last she was released, I picked her up and drove her home. I don't remember seeing her much after that, but Joe continued to visit her. When Joe

---

‡   See the Resources section at the end of this book (page 287).

was eventually elected mayor, I heard from another client that Gloria enjoyed bragging that she was friends with the mayor.

Sometimes, caring for our pets takes a village.

After Rana and I returned home from the hospital, my doctor side resurfaced, reminding me that I did have resources I could access. I had the oncologists at Tufts. I had my colleagues at the clinic, and Dr. LeVan, the veterinary dentist. I had my medical training, which gave me the tools to evaluate medical articles and concepts. And I had my recent training in TCVM. In addition, I had the support of friends and family, including Mike and Lisa.

As it turned out, I would need all the resources at my disposal and then some to care for Rana.

11

He Knew Just What to Do

As Rana's diagnosis was unfolding, I realized that something else was happening in the household: Daiquiri, my cat, had stopped eating.

For the first couple of days, I was so distraught about Rana that I barely realized what was going on. Next, I concluded he must be reacting to my sadness and stress. After a few more days, however, I realized something could be seriously wrong.

Daiquiri was a cat who *always* ate. He would eat the house, I liked to joke. Now, he wouldn't touch his food. My sweet kitty was sixteen years old, but of course I hoped he would live several more years, into the far reaches of his possible life expectancy.

I drew some blood from him and sent it off to the lab. When I received the results, I understood why he wasn't eating. His liver was failing.

I made an appointment to bring Daiquiri out to the clinic for an ultrasound the following day. That morning, I woke up and sat with my cat. I listened to my intuition, and I reached a conclusion. My cat was not going to come back from this illness. The ultrasound would be for me, not for him. It would only confirm what he and I already knew. I canceled the appointment. Daiquiri had enjoyed a miraculous recovery a year earlier, but this time, it felt as though he was telling me not to try.

Daiquiri took up residence in the half bathroom on the second floor, a tiny but peaceful space with no windows. It was a place he had never hung out in before—why would he? It was a half bath. But there he was, curled up on the floor in front of the sink. I tried to bring him into the bedroom or downstairs into the living room or the kitchen to be with us, but he just found his way back upstairs to the half bath. Eventually, I sat with him there.

I saw acceptance in my cat's eyes as I watched him slowly fade, and though I struggled with the pain of losing him, I was comforted by his serenity. He purred as I stroked his head. I offered him everything I could think of to eat, but he continued to politely refuse. He was calm and seemed at peace. I took my cues from him. Daiquiri knew he was dying, and he was okay with it. He knew just what to do. I thanked him for being the best cat ever, and gazed into his beautiful iridescent green eyes. I told him how much I loved him, and that I understood he needed to leave, that I would let him go, and he didn't have to stay for me.

Lisa later told me that on the day of the surgeon's phone call about Rana, she had gone upstairs and had her own conversation with Daiquiri. She asked him not to leave just yet, but to try to hang on for a couple more days. And he did.

Each day, I kept Daiquiri company, there on the bathroom floor, reliving all our time together. Finally, after a few days, I decided it was time to intervene. His skin was yellowed from jaundice, and he was weak. He still did not seem uncomfortable, but I felt it was the right time.

I called Eileen. She told me she would be at the clinic the follow-ing morning, a Sunday, caring for hospitalized animal patients and would be able to euthanize my sweet kitty there. We agreed that I would give him a tranquilizer injection at home, so he would not be awake for the car ride. He would then pass peacefully at the clinic.

I could have euthanized Daiquiri by myself, of course, either at home or at the clinic. But with my own animal, I didn't want to focus on the needle going into the vein. I didn't want to think about logistics. I wanted to be fully present in the last moments of my friend's life.

I wanted to be a client.

Sunday morning was Mother's Day. I whispered loving words to my cat as I injected the tiny needle with the tranquilizer into the muscle of his back leg. Mike drove to the clinic while I held Daiquiri in my arms. Inside, we waited in a private room for Eileen, who had not yet arrived at the clinic. We waited a long time. Even-tually the receptionist came in—Eileen was on the phone. Her kids had surprised her with breakfast in bed, she told me. She would be in very soon, and she apologized for keeping me waiting.

I imagined how torn Eileen was, wanting to enjoy the special time with her children, knowing her friend and colleague was wait-ing for her at the clinic with her dying cat. I felt guilty, placing her in that situation.

Finally, Eileen arrived. I assured her I understood why she was late. By this time, Daiquiri was starting to wake up from the tran-quilizer. I felt bad that he was waking up, and I stroked his fur and spoke to him as Eileen gave the final injection.

My sweet, sweet kitty. My first cat. Daiquiri.

Later, I concluded that Daiquiri chose the time during Rana's diagnosis because he wanted to slip away in the background. He was that type of kitty.

Daiquiri's illness fit a pattern I had learned was common, es-pecially for cats: to appear physically healthy and then suddenly succumb to a severe illness. I'd even come up with a name for this pattern: the "he was fine on Tuesday" cat. I noticed early on in my career that I would sometimes see a cat who was very ill, yet the owners would claim the cat had been "fine on Tuesday" (or a few days ago, last week, or whatever). I was not normally skeptical of what my clients told me, but this didn't seem to add up. These cats had clearly been sick for some time. Often the cat would have a chronic illness, a condition I knew had not started only a few days earlier. At first, I concluded that perhaps these cats kept to themselves, or maybe some cat owners were not very observant. Eventually, though, I heard the "fine on Tuesday" claim from enough clients I knew to be observant, highly capable cat owners that I decided to rethink what was going on. If these people told me their cat was eating, playing, and purring normally on Tuesday, I believed them. What was happening, then?

Cats, I finally realized, are extremely good at hiding their illnesses, even from devoted and attentive caretakers. Weight loss may be the only early symptom, and chronic weight loss is difficult to observe when you see an animal daily. Other than that, these cats acted normally. One theory is that they do this because in the wild, if they exhibit weakness, they are more likely to become prey. Another possibility is that even with a serious illness, they feel well, until suddenly they don't.

As hard as it is to lose a pet to a sudden illness, I have often reminded clients that it is something many of us would wish for ourselves. To live (hopefully) a long life, and to feel well until the end of it, is a blessing, as hard as it is for those who are left behind.

I was comforted to know that Daiquiri had enjoyed a long and healthy life (although not as long as I had hoped), as well as a peaceful passing, but I still ached for him. It felt like the end of an era. Daiquiri and I had been together since my first week of veterinary school, during what felt like my entire adult life.

And now I had to face Rana's illness without his support.

12

Go Toward

As I mourned my cat, I struggled to understand the reason for Rana's illness, so unusual in such a young dog. I couldn't seem to accept that such a thing was possible, and it seemed to change my whole worldview. Of course, I knew that bad things happen and that life can be unfair. But I couldn't seem to accept that *this thing* was happening. I kept thinking about her young age, and the fact that she was a mixed-breed dog; the combination of both factors making a cancer diagnosis statistically extremely unlikely. There are certain breeds more prone to cancers, among them boxers, golden retrievers, and flat-coated retrievers. But mixed-breed dogs tend to be healthier in general due to something called hybrid vigor—the mixing of the gene pool makes it less likely that the animals will inherit genetic issues.

As a pet owner, I struggled to understand. What caused the cancer? Could she have gotten into something toxic and carcinogenic before I met her? Did I miss something in my care of her? Could

I have prevented this? If only I had brushed her teeth regularly, I chided myself, perhaps I would have noticed the tumor sooner.

I reminded myself of the countless times I had answered similar questions for others as a medical professional. I've assured many people that their pet's cancer had not resulted from something they'd either done or failed to do.

"That's the sixty-four-million-dollar question" was my stock response when asked what causes cancer. Then I would discuss what we knew: many cancers have multiple causes, including possible genetic factors.

I knew that people often blamed themselves after a pet's cancer diagnosis; it was something I had witnessed over and over. I had a wonderful older kitty patient named Blackie, who had a devoted owner named Laurie. One day, Laurie called me to come and have a look at Blackie. Laurie felt his appetite had decreased, and she had noticed he was drooling a bit. She thought perhaps he was suffering from an abscessed tooth. When I arrived at the house and examined Blackie, I noticed a slight asymmetry to his lower jaw. As soon as I put my hands on the area, I could tell it was a tumor and not an abscess; the area felt firm and hard. A look in his mouth confirmed my suspicions. Reluctantly, I explained my findings to Laurie.

"I can't believe I didn't notice it," she said, shaking her head. "I should have seen it before. I'm not a good owner."

I had known Laurie for many years and seen firsthand the excellent care she had provided for her beloved Blackie. "Laurie, you are not a veterinarian with over twenty years of experience," I reminded her. "You called me as soon as you noticed a problem. There is nothing you could have done to prevent this or to have seen it sooner." I was glad she had voiced her concerns so I could talk to her and explain that Blackie could not have had a better or more loving owner.

———————

As all these thoughts were floating through my head, I remember sensing that I had an important decision to make. This was not a decision about Rana's care, but about my feelings for her. I felt a need to formally decide how to proceed emotionally.

One option, I felt, would be to start to emotionally detach from her, knowing she had a terminal disease. This would probably be the prudent choice. Alternatively, I could continue to feel the same way toward her and maintain the status quo.

A third option arose in my mind as a whisper: *Go toward.*

To go toward Rana, knowing she would die young, would be to fully commit to her, allowing my emotions free rein. It would be to fully embrace the time we had left together.

I chose to go toward.

I wish I could say I was stoic, but I was a wreck. Unless I was at work, I cried constantly, overcome by the thought of life without Rana. I couldn't seem to wrap my mind around what was happening. I knew how I wanted to feel, which was to be in the moment, mindfully enjoying the time I still had with my precious dog. But that feeling seemed out of reach.

Mike tried to help. One day I went into the kitchen to find the Serenity Prayer taped to the fridge:

Grant me the serenity
To accept the things I cannot change,
The courage to change the things I can,
And the wisdom to know the difference.

I believed in the words, but I couldn't seem to translate them into my heart. I read them daily, yet they remained just words.

I cried when I was in the car alone, when I snuggled with Rana, when I woke up in the morning, and when I couldn't sleep at night.

My husband was exhausted from trying to console me all the time, as well as from dealing with his own sadness. At one point he said, "She's only a dog!"

I stared at him, sensing his frustration. Fortunately, I recognized this for what it was: his supportive strategies were not working, so he figured he would try something new. "No!" I wailed. "Tough love is NOT what I need right now!"

I had an annual physical exam coming up; I decided to ask my physician for antidepressants. At my appointment, my doctor—a dog lover—listened intently, sympathetically. I told her I didn't *want* antidepressants, but I was having trouble functioning. My doctor was nodding and writing out a prescription before I finished my story. By the weekend, I had stopped crying. I felt a peculiar numbness. But it was better than the constant pain.

Whenever I looked at Rana, all I could think about was losing her. I didn't know it then, but what I was feeling was common, and there is even a name for it: anticipatory grief.

Now that I know what it is called, I can recognize it, and I see it often.

Barry had been my patient since he was a young adult. My assistant Michelle and I couldn't help wanting to play with the happy, rambunctious dog whenever he came in for a clinic visit.

When Barry was about seven years old, his owner Kathy brought him in to see me and began to cry. Barry was fine, she said, but she had recently learned that two of his littermates had died of cancer within the past year. She and I both knew that flat-coated retrievers were very prone to cancer and many dogs succumbed in middle age.

I examined Barry and told her he appeared to be in excellent health; although he had mellowed from his excitable puppy stage, he practically glowed with happiness and energy. However, Kathy and I both knew there were no guarantees about how long he would live. She didn't have a diagnosis for Barry, yet she was distraught at the mere thought of losing him. I consoled her as much as I could.

Animals have such short lives, and as a veterinarian, I know all too well how easily we can lose our animal friends. One day, I sat on the love seat with Rana, looking out at the lake, thinking about the mysteries of time. She was here, now; it seemed impossible that someday soon, she wouldn't be.

It has been reported that many dogs do not like to be hugged. Hugs mean something different to dogs than they do to humans; while a hug does constitute a physical touch, to put pressure over the back of a dog's neck and shoulders is something a dominant dog will do, or a mother dog to a puppy. However, some dogs do enjoy what we call hugs, and Rana was one of them. She was a sucker for physical touch. She loved to cuddle, loved to lie with her head on my foot, loved to be patted, have her paws held, smoosh her head into me, and have her ears (very) gently pulled.

On that day, I hugged Rana as we sat together. I knew she understood I was in pain and upset; she was always trying to comfort me. She snuggled and leaned into me, and I yearned to pause time. *I am going to stay here, and this hug will go on for all eternity. I'll hold her here and I will not let go. I will not let go of this dog. I will stop time during this hug.*

We remained there for a long, long time. Eventually, of course, we separated. But it's a memory that has sustained me, and I think of it still. In some dimension, Rana and I are still hugging, there on the love seat, looking out over the lake.

13

Bucket List

The next step for Rana was to meet with the radiation oncologist at Tufts, to see whether they could offer anything to help her, as surgery was now out of the question. I scheduled the appointment, and Lisa volunteered to come with me. Together we sat in the waiting room at Tufts. I was familiar with the waiting room of an animal hospital, but only as a doctor or a veterinary student. I was not used to sitting there, worrying about my pet, waiting to hear her name called.

Lisa tried to distract me. "Check out that woman over there. She matches her dog!" she whispered. The woman, holding the leash of a black-and-white springer spaniel, was dressed entirely in black and white.

When we were finally called into the exam room, Lisa pulled out a notebook and took notes as I spoke to the doctor, in case I forgot anything that was said.

The radiation oncologist was sympathetic, but the news she had for me was grim.

"Your dog has about a three-month prognosis with no treatment. With radiation, she might have eight months," she told me. However, the radiation oncologist went on to explain that if Rana were to have the type of radiation on her face she was recommending, she would not be able to run off leash, or swim, for several weeks.

"What about chemotherapy?" I asked. I looked over at Lisa, who grimaced sympathetically and continued writing.

"Rana's type of tumor is not one that tends to metastasize, or spread. Instead, it is very locally invasive. Right now, we don't have a chemo protocol for her condition."

"What will . . . happen as the tumor grows?" I asked.

"Her mouth will become painful, and she will probably stop eating," she answered. "She may begin to paw at her mouth."

"When will this happen?" I closed my eyes.

"I think that in about a month, you will notice her having pain in her mouth."

I looked over at Rana, who was enjoying the attention, although she may have been confused by the sad atmosphere in the room. Eventually all my questions were answered, and Lisa and I gathered our things and walked out of the animal hospital with Rana, into the warm spring sunshine.

As the fog of information cleared, it became an easy decision. I wanted to make the rest of Rana's life as wonderful as possible. If my dog had only one summer left, she was going to spend it swimming and running off leash, I concluded. She was going to chase ducks until they flew away. I was not going to take that away from her, not even to increase my precious time with her. Mike and Lisa agreed.

I also realized I did have more options. At the time, I had not treated any animals with cancer holistically, but I knew many veterinarians did. I contacted my favorite acupuncture teacher, Dr. Steve

Marsden, again. He was coming to Tufts soon to teach a workshop; perhaps he would be able to examine Rana. Steve, I reminded myself, was the reason Daiquiri had lived an extra year.

Once again, Steve was generous with his time and spoke to me at length. We talked about diet, supplements, and Chinese herbal formulas.

After my conversation with Steve, I felt like I was on a mission. I threw myself into Rana's care. He had recommended a home-cooked diet with ground-up raw vegetables. This, I could do. However, although I enjoyed cooking, I had always been intimidated by food processors and didn't own one. If I was looking through a cookbook or a magazine and saw a recipe for something appealing, as soon as I noticed a food processor was involved, I turned the page. It was a deal-breaker. Now, I would need one to prepare the diet Steve recommended.

"You can borrow mine," said my friend Janet. "I hardly ever use it."

The food processor arrived with a paper bag full of scary-looking attachments and gizmos that I promptly packed away out of sight on a shelf by the washing machine. I read the manual for the food processor, determined to conquer my phobia. Janet had shown me which blade to use and assured me I was quite capable of operating the machine.

At the supermarket I bought all kinds of vegetables for Rana— kale, spinach, broccoli, cauliflower, and sprouts. I bought meat to cook for her. I also obtained several supplements, and bonemeal for calcium. Then I got to work. I cooked the meat, ground the vegetables, mixed and measured the supplements. Later, I placed some of Rana's newly prepared food in her bowl, along with some of her old food, to give her a gradual transition that would not upset her digestive system.

I was not prepared for the feeling that came over me when I put the bowl of food down and Rana started to eat. *I had done this for her*—I had prepared her food myself, with love and care. It was the first time during this ordeal I felt there was something I could do. I hadn't realized how helpless I'd been feeling until I watched Rana eat the food I had prepared with my own hands. If cooking for my dog was going to help her, then I was all in.

Previously, I had thought people who cooked for their pets were a little strange or perhaps had too much time on their hands. I often didn't have the time or the energy to cook for myself and my husband, never mind an animal. Yet now I was not only doing it but enjoying it. Preparing Rana's food seemed to help me as much as it helped her. Rana had always loved to eat, but she especially adored the home-cooked food. I felt a swell of pleasure every time I fed her.

When Steve arrived at Tufts to teach his seminar a month or so later, he suggested I bring Rana in for him to examine in front of the class as a case study. We gathered in a lounge area with sofas so everyone could watch closely. Standing on the couch cushions, Rana enjoyed the attention. I patted my dog's head as Steve felt her pulse. "Hmm," he said, "let's try this." He inserted a single needle into an acupuncture point near her knee. Rana's response was dramatic; her entire body relaxed and she nearly fell off the sofa. We all laughed. Once again, I was amazed at Steve's expertise. He recommended some Chinese herbs for Rana based on his findings, and I smiled in relief.

Rana responded well to her new diet, which was low in carbohydrates, and to the herbs and supplements. She lost a little body fat, and her muscles seemed more defined. Her coat was glossy and smooth. At a house call, I described how she looked to a client, who responded, "You mean she looks buff!" I agreed. Rana was looking buff.

Mike helped a lot with Rana's food preparation. Although I did learn how to use the food processor, Mike took over the job, mostly to free up my time for assembling Rana's many medications and supplements—Lisa had found some little plastic containers at a yard sale, and I used them for pill containers. Mike and I found we could grind about five to six days' worth of vegetables in advance (although we learned that cauliflower gets a bit stinky by day five). Sometimes we would have enough food for ourselves in the fridge but would need to go the store because Rana needed more food. Mike, a vegetarian at the time, was surprised by how easily he had adapted to buying and cooking meat for a dog. I was not surprised. He had come to love her just as intensely as I did. It was a bitter-sweet feeling to watch him dote on her, knowing her illness had drawn them closer together.

Rana's tumor continued to grow. I watched as it spread from the right side of her upper gum, across the front of her mouth, and over to the left side. Soon, part of her gum was protruding from her mouth. Her incisor teeth, the small teeth in the front of a dog's mouth, separated as the gum widened and enlarged. Still, she seemed to feel no pain. Rana continued to eat, and Mike and I continued to cook.

One weekend, we brought the dogs to Maine to visit Karen and her husband, Tom. Karen was also stunned by Rana's diagnosis. At her parents' lake house, Karen waded into the water with her camera, positioning herself to catch photos of Rana as she leaped off the dock for tennis balls. I was amazed at how happy my dog was; her spirit was as bright as ever.

I had always thought Rana would make a great agility dog, and that she would enjoy learning it. Dog agility is a sport in which dogs run through obstacle courses consisting of jumps, hoops, ramps, tunnels, and seesaws. Training a dog to enjoy an agility course involves plenty of treats and positive reinforcement, and it fosters an intimate working relationship between human and dog.

After Rana's diagnosis, I decided to sign the two of us up for a series of agility classes, as soon as possible. A receptionist at the clinic recommended a place about a twenty-five-minute drive away, with a well-known teacher and a large indoor arena, and I made the arrangements.

At the first class, Rana and I and the other human-dog teams learned clicker training. I had attended a clicker training talk at a veterinary conference some years before by one of the pioneers of clicker training, Karen Pryor. I'd been extremely impressed with the talk (which included a video of a clicker-trained goldfish, among other animals) and had bought Dr. Pryor's book. I found the psychology behind clicker training fascinating.

First, we had to "load" the clicker, which meant we had to teach our dogs that the clicker noise means food is coming. Once the dogs learned that, it became easier to shape their behavior and get them to do precisely what you are asking them to do. Behavior shaping was a concept I remembered from my college psychology class.

Next, we needed to familiarize the dogs with the various equipment in the room. Rana was interested in everything and unafraid of the obstacles. She enjoyed the agility class and was good at it, just as I had thought she would be.

During one class, the teacher, Betty, noticed I was looking downcast. She knew about Rana's cancer and her poor prognosis.

"Rana's going to live forever," she told me firmly, in her no-nonsense voice. "Let's try her on this obstacle over here." I tried to smile, warmed by her kindness.

Betty also gave Rana some surprising praise. "She's really smart!" she commented one day. I almost burst out laughing. Poor Rana; Mike and I tended to compare her to her housemate Trudy, who was extremely intelligent. Rana was known in our home for her cuteness, not her smarts. But Betty was an experienced dog trainer who didn't mince words. If she said Rana was smart, she was smart!

One evening, at our second to last class, Rana and I were both tired. It had been a hot day, and I had squeezed into my schedule an emergency euthanasia for one of my patients, an older kitty who had suddenly failed. The procedure had gone well, but of course, it was sad. My dinner had consisted of a peanut butter sandwich in the car on the way to agility class. During the last ten minutes of the class, Rana was running on a low balance beam, and I was running next to her, holding her leash. Suddenly, from the middle of the beam, Rana jumped right in front of me. It took me by surprise, and my legs tangled together as I fell forward over her body. Rana was fine, but my foot and ankle hurt terribly.

The owner of the facility ran and got me a bucket of ice water so I could submerge my foot. I felt stupid; I must not have been paying attention. After fifteen minutes or so of keeping my foot submerged in the ice bucket as much as I could, I tried to stand. And collapsed. By now it was after 9:00 p.m. Although I had injured my left foot, there was no way I could drive because it was so painful. I had to call Mike at home, as he was getting ready for bed, and tell him he needed to come and pick us up, drop Rana off at home, and bring me to the hospital.

At the emergency room, the good news was that nothing appeared to be broken. What I had was an awfully bad sprain of both my foot and my ankle. I went home on crutches.

"No more agility class for you," said my husband.

I needed the crutches for about ten days, after which I was able to use a cane. I went to physical therapy twice a week. My ankle and foot remained painful, and recovery was slow.

When I returned to work at the clinic the week after my injury, a technician gave me a stool to sit on and a bell to ring if I needed assistance. "You'll be all right," she said. "This is what we did after Dr. Smith broke her foot."

I called in my first client from the waiting room. After I announced the dog's name, a man stood up, holding the leash of a young active pointer. My discomfort must have shown in my face, because as the client walked in, he asked doubtfully, "Should you be working?"

"I'm okay," I responded, trying not to wince. "It's not broken. Just sprained." I smiled bravely.

"What did you do to yourself?" he asked, trying to prevent his dog from knocking me over. I realized I would have to ring for assistance. It was going to be a long day.

"Oh, well, actually I fell over my dog. At, uh . . . at agility class," I responded sheepishly. "*Dog* agility class."

14

Dances with Death

Veterinarians have an unusual relationship with our patients' mortality, as along with working to help animals live, we sometimes help them die. Like our human physician counterparts, we spend a good part of our time trying to stave off death, through preventive care, vaccinations, and care of severely ill and hurt animals; we do all we can to prevent and alleviate suffering. On the other hand, unlike physicians, we are regularly—sometimes daily—called upon to alleviate suffering through euthanasia.

As a veterinary student, I had struggled with the concept of it, and how easy it was to summon Death to end the life of a patient.

Death seems to respect me, for he always responds to my requests for him to arrive, I journaled as a new graduate. At times he will arrive unbidden, and he and I will struggle over a creature . . . It is part of my job to dance with Death. People come to me to ask me to be a link for their animals, either to prevent Death, or to welcome him.

In other words, euthanasia kind of creeped me out. When I

performed one, it felt as though I had been given privileged access to a special power I didn't understand, that nobody understood. I didn't know what to make of it.

While we did have an ethics class in veterinary school, the focus was mainly on legal situations. We were taught it would be unethical (and likely illegal) to agree to euthanize a client's animal and instead find it another home without their permission, even if the animal was young and healthy. We did not discuss what it would *feel like* to euthanize an animal. I still remember a dog I treated as a new graduate that had been hit by a car. My patient was in physiologic shock, which I threw myself into treating, managing to keep her alive. When she was stable, X-rays revealed that her pelvis was shattered, and her owners elected to euthanize her. Just hours after saving her life, I ended it. It was the first time, but not the last, that I had to swing from one extreme to the other on the same animal on the same day.

Many people, including myself, get upset if a dog dies in a movie or a book; this is such a common phenomenon that a website exists called Doesthedogdie.com. The site has a searchable database of spoilers and content warnings for dozens of categories, all added after the initial category of death of a canine. But as a veterinarian, it's not something I can avoid.

When I was new to performing euthanasia, it was the taking of a life that was challenging for me. I was amazed by how a simple intravenous injection could wield such enormous power over life and death. What *was* life, if you could end it so easily? At home, I regarded my own pets differently, knowing how little it would take for them to die.

As time went by, I became more accustomed to the concept. Many animals I euthanized were within days of dying on their own, others were uncomfortable and suffering. I often felt I was performing an ethically honorable task: something my mother terms a mitzvah, a Hebrew word meaning a good deed, a sacred duty in the Jewish faith.

People sometimes ask whether a pet should view the body of a deceased animal housemate. I believe this is a good idea, although I also think the remaining animal usually already knows that its family member was ill, both by the sick pet's behavior and by its smell.

I once performed an at-home euthanasia for a dog named Sal. The owners had placed their other dog, Louie, in a separate room while I euthanized the sick dog. After Sal died, they went to retrieve Louie. I sat on the side of the room farthest from the door, next to Sal's body. As Louie entered the room, he raised his head and sniffed the air. Then his entire body language changed. He knew instantly, likely from a smell indistinguishable to the human nose, that Sal had died. In that situation, many humans would likely approach the body, needing to look closely or even to touch the deceased animal to realize death had occurred. I have rarely seen an animal do that. They appear to gather this information from several feet away. Animals understand death far more than we give them credit for—and, quite possibly, better than people.

At the clinic one day, the receptionist handed me a patient's chart and asked if I could do a euthanasia. It was scheduled for the other doctor, but she was backed up with an emergency, and the client didn't have a preference regarding which doctor performed the procedure. Euthanasia often happens with no time for a doctor to mentally prepare. It's not uncommon for an appointment with a very sick or injured animal to end with euthanasia.

I entered the exam room and found a middle-aged woman and her teenage daughter sitting on the floor. The patient, a very old kitty named Cleo, was wrapped in a towel in the woman's lap.

I sat on the floor with them. This is how a euthanasia begins for me, with getting onto the client's level as best I can. Sometimes it is a client and a pet I know well, and sometimes they are complete strangers.

I stroked Cleo's head and remarked upon how soft and beautiful her fur was. I gently asked the client how Cleo had been doing lately, and she described a lack of appetite, vomiting, and general discomfort. I noticed the wasted muscles, the protrusion of bones on the cat's body. We talked about what a wonderful pet she had been and what a long life she had enjoyed. Both the woman and her daughter seemed comfortable with Cleo being euthanized.

Next, I asked if they had ever witnessed a euthanasia before. It's a question I often ask, and my purpose is to gauge the owner's comfort level with what is about to happen. It's an opportunity for the person to let me know if they are nervous, so I can give them some additional reassurance and answer any questions they may have.

I explained that the injection is a painless overdose of anesthetic, but I felt Cleo would be more comfortable if I gave her a tranquilizer injection first, so she wouldn't be stressed when I placed the tourniquet on her leg and gave the intravenous injection. I told them Cleo's eyes would likely stay open, and she might urinate and defecate afterward as her muscles relaxed. I explained that I would check Cleo's heart to make sure she was gone and that they mustn't worry if they saw any twitches or muscle spasms. I let them know that, after the procedure, they could stay in the room with Cleo for as long as they liked.

Cleo barely noticed the tranquilizer injection and shortly afterward placed her head down in the woman's lap as she lost consciousness. I gently picked up Cleo's front paw and shaved some fur so I could visualize her vein. I set the fur aside on Cleo's towel and told her people that, if they wanted, they could take it home as a keepsake (many owners appreciate this, although some comment wryly that they have plenty of fur at home).

Next, I placed the rubber tourniquet around Cleo's front leg and tightened it. I put alcohol on the leg to better see Cleo's vein. I made my silent prayer that all would go smoothly for Cleo and her family, setting my intention of doing my best for them. And I inserted the tiny needle into her vein. When I knew the needle was in place, I released the tourniquet and began injecting the euthanasia solution.

Just as I gave the injection, Cleo's owner looked at me with moist eyes. "This must be so hard for you," she said.

I was stunned by her compassion, at the very moment of her cat's death.

Yet I was unable to admit the truth even to myself. I didn't say, "Yes, it's hard to bear witness to so much love, so much gratitude, so much grief." I didn't say, "I feel a lot of pressure for things to go smoothly" or "I can never allow my emotions to interfere with my work."

Instead, I told a small lie.

I said, "I only do it when I believe it is the right thing to do."

Cleo died peacefully. When the injection was finished, I withdrew the needle, carefully placing a cotton ball over the leg to catch any bleeding. I put my stethoscope on and listened for Cleo's heartbeat. I heard only the gentle rustle of the heart's contents as the blood settled and came to rest.

"She's gone," I said softly after a moment. We all stroked Cleo's soft fur and told her what a good kitty she'd been.

"She's so peaceful," her owner observed quietly.

"Yes," I replied, "people often say that. They really do look peaceful."

Most veterinarians have heard the statement uttered by Cleo's owner countless times. Even more common is the statement, "I would love to be a veterinarian, but I know I could *never* put an animal to sleep." People mean well, and are often grateful, yet it's an isolating feeling to be told repeatedly that a critical element of your work is unimaginable.

Which is probably why I lie.

My statement to Cleo's owner, *I only do it when I believe it's the right thing to do*, is something I've repeated to myself as well as to clients. It is mostly true. It is often true. But it is not always true. In addition to the healthy shelter dogs I euthanized early in my career, I have euthanized clients' animals that could have lived if they were treated. Faced with a sick or injured animal the client can't afford or doesn't want to treat, I ask myself, would this animal be adoptable? Typically the answer is no. And because I'm aware that even healthy adoptable animals are euthanized at shelters every day, I am able, however unhappily, to proceed with a difficult and emotionally painful task.

This is the reason I will always adopt from rescues or shelters. I couldn't save those lives, but I will save other ones.

Eventually I grew accustomed to the process of ending a life through euthanasia. It was a bit like adjusting to performing surgery—how strange did it feel, initially, to have my hands (gloved, of course) inside the body of one of my patients? To see and feel their internal organs, to cut and sew tissue and skin? It took some getting used to. After a while, surgery was just another day at the office.

Euthanasia, however, is unique. For myself and, I imagine, most veterinarians, there will never be "just another euthanasia." Each one entails being fully present, as a sign of respect—for life, for death, for the individual being, for their human family. If the owner is not present for the procedure I can focus all my attention on the animal. I am always conscious of the fact that my voice will be the last voice the animal hears, and my touch will be the last touch; I am aware that the veterinary assistant or technician holding the animal feels the same way. We don't speak about this, but it is always the case, no matter who I am working with.

If the animal's owner is present, I experience another dimension of awareness: I am hypersensitive to the person's emotional state. I know that the same act I perform to relieve an animal's pain can cause profound suffering on the part of their human family.

Part of the reason I adjusted to performing euthanasia was the patients themselves. Animals, I have come to believe, do not fear death as most people do. They try to avoid it, certainly. Like humans, they have a survival instinct, which can be fierce. Yet when I see animals in the process of dying, they seem to experience a calm acceptance. And by *acceptance*, I do not mean resignation; I mean recognition and acknowledgment. I mean a true, full comprehension of mortality.

The time surrounding death, for animals, is less of a cerebral experience and more of an intuitive, instinctual one. Many of the animals I euthanize are gravely ill and would likely die within a matter of days, or sometimes hours. These animals, I believe, know their death is near, and they are not afraid. The reason is this: they realize their body is breaking down. They know, as do other animals in the household, that they are dying. This is something they don't think about *before* their body is failing. But when it is *actually happening*, they can interpret and accept this knowledge. Much as the cat Snowball adjusted to the loss of her leg, animals near death recognize an internal process outside their control. They make appropriate adjustments, such as hiding or not eating. They trust the intuition that has helped them all their lives as they receive messages from their physical body.

How can you possibly know that? you might ask; perhaps it is simply a story you tell yourself, as you attempt to comprehend something essentially incomprehensible or to assuage some hidden guilt. *Well,* I might respond, *I spend a lot of time with animals.* They are my teachers, and I believe this to be true: many animals experience a profound mind-body connection as they are dying. My best teacher was my own cat, Daiquiri.

Perhaps he was special, you might reply, *an exception.*

And I would tell you that I have seen his wisdom, his knowledge and acceptance of death, reflected in many other eyes.

Dogs and cats may be skilled at hiding pain, but fear is an emotion visible to those of us who work with them. Some of the animals I see every day are anxious, apprehensive, even afraid. I work hard to reassure them, distract them, and calm them. Reading fear is a part of my job, and not only for the sake of my patients. A fearful animal may claw or bite, sometimes without warning. I assess fear to protect myself, my veterinary technician and assistant coworkers, and my clients from serious injury.

Among the near-death animals I have attended, I have occasionally sensed a reluctance to leave their people, and anxiety over my presence or about being in a hospital, but I have not seen what I would term *fear* as an animal is dying.

This may be why I don't personally fear death. It's not that I want to die. I don't, and a part of me doesn't expect to, because it's unfathomable. And though I'm not afraid of death, I am afraid of suffering, and of watching others suffer, and of knowing my death is imminent and unavoidable due to a tragic accident or violence. But death itself? When people say they fear death, it confuses me. I hope to avoid death for a long time, to live a long and happy and fulfilling life, and to die peacefully. When I am in the process of dying, my physical body breaking down, I may not want to leave it, but I also hope to recognize what is happening and to acknowledge the inevitable process on a deeper level, as I have seen so many animals do.

After I began doing house calls, people who were not my clients started to call and ask me to euthanize their pet at home. I was hesitant at first, but their requests made sense, especially after they explained how nervous their pet became at the veterinary clinic and how important it was to them that their beloved companion was not anxious in his or her final moments.

I understood. I wouldn't want to be anxious in my last moments, either.

Home euthanasia often seemed a better experience for the clients as well as the pet. People could focus on their pet without the added distraction of other clients and animals, ringing phones, barking dogs, and the general hubbub of a veterinary clinic. Other than my presence, they could enjoy the privacy and familiar comfort of their own home. And they didn't have to drive afterward. I have worried many times about distraught people driving after their beloved pet has died or been euthanized.

However, entering a stranger's home and meeting them for the first time, to facilitate an intense, emotionally painful, and private moment in their lives, was not easy. At first, I struggled to feel comfortable. As with regular house calls, I was not in control of the environment. I had no support staff and couldn't leave the room if I wanted to take a minute to mentally regroup. I needed to remain fully present, no matter how challenging the experience.

As I drove to a house-call euthanasia, I could feel myself preparing for the task ahead of me. It was different from driving to a regular appointment. As I drew closer to the client's address, I'd turn off the radio or change from my typical soft rock or NPR station to classical music.

Once I entered the client's home, it was up to me to read people's cues and set them at ease. Some people wanted to tell stories about their pet. Some needed to make sure I agreed with their decision to euthanize, while others were already emotionally committed to the procedure and didn't require any further discussion. Some wanted to fully concentrate on their animal, while others were anxious; if I sensed this I would try to keep up a stream of conversation to help distract them (this tended to be the case if the television was on when I arrived).

Some people wanted to make sure I agreed that euthanasia was warranted, especially if the animal happened to be having a good day. "I almost called you to cancel because she ate a bit this morning and took a few steps," a client may confide. Once I confirm that euthanasia is still reasonable, I'll remind the owner that it's not a bad thing if the last day is a good day.

There may be only one person present or a larger audience, including adult children and their significant others. I've seen divorced couples reunite to bid farewell to the pet they'd adopted together. Emotions run high, and family members may bicker with one another, which is understandable but still makes me feel awkward.

I'll perform the procedure right where the animal was resting as I entered the home, or on a bed or a sofa, or in the owner's arms. Others ask to have the euthanasia done outdoors, perhaps near a favorite spot in the yard. Some people light incense, show me photos, feed their pet a favorite food if they are still able to eat.

No two euthanasia procedures are ever the same.

The words spoken to a dying pet at the moment of euthanasia are some of the most beautiful words I have ever heard. *I love you* is the most common sentiment, followed by *thank you*.

I love you so much.
Thank you for being there for me when my mother died.
You are the best dog ever.
Say hi to Papa and Dusty and Comet for me.

My job is not simply the giving of an injection, or an explanation, or a hug. The craftwork happens in the emotional and perhaps spiritual space between the animal, the person, and me. The gift I receive is a glimpse into the bond between human and animal. It feels as though, for a moment, I can experience the connection between them; perhaps a tiny bit of that connection becomes a part of me. It is a privilege, but like many privileges, it comes with its own burden. Sometimes I find it hard to reenter my own life. It's as though a part of me remains there, in the space between human and animal, life and death.

Occasionally, if there are only myself and one other person alone in a quiet room, I'll notice something as or just after I give the euthanasia injection. I think of it as a sea change, a profound change in the environment around me. The main things I sense are a change in the light and, sometimes, the sound of wind in the trees. It feels as though there has been a shift in the room. A presence that was there is now gone. I am conscious of a sense of peace, of connection; I am in a state of meditative awe. While I haven't noticed any physical changes to my patient in these moments, I can *feel* that the animal has died. The body may be present, but the spirit has left the room.

Once the euthanasia solution has been administered and the animal's breathing stops, it can take a few minutes for the heart to stop beating, especially in a sick, geriatric animal who may have poor circulation. I'd rather avoid telling a distraught client that their pet still has a faint heartbeat and that I'll need to listen again in a few minutes to make sure their animal is truly deceased. So I'll move slowly afterward. I'll sit for a moment, reflecting or talking with the owner, before moving to put on my stethoscope. When I feel a sea change, I *know* the animal has died. I still put on my stethoscope and listen carefully for heart sounds. Yet my mental state is different. Rather than hoping enough time has passed, I am secure in the knowledge that it has.

I don't always feel a sea change. I'm more likely to notice it when there is silence in the room, when neither I nor the owner(s) are speaking. Perhaps I am more able to be fully present. Whatever the reason, when it does happen, the ending of a life feels to me like a meditation.

15

A New Addition

I was reluctant to leave Rana at all after her diagnosis. Mike and I had planned to bring her with us on a camping weekend that summer, and the problem was how to manage her food during the trip. Rana continued to eat with gusto, and I was loath to make any changes, even for a few days. By then, she was taking several herbs and supplements, and I had become almost superstitious about them, not wanting her to miss any of her medications, not even for a day. In hindsight, I wasn't quite rational about it. But then, nothing about Rana seemed rational; not her diagnosis, not how well she was doing, nor my feelings for her. And while I may look back and think I was being a bit ridiculous or too controlling, at the time it seemed vitally important that I adhere precisely to her dietary regimen. I was afraid if I interfered with one strand, the fragile web keeping Rana alive would collapse.

So Mike and I sat down to plan. We were going for three days, and we would need six meals. We would need to have all her vegetables ground ahead of time, so we would need to bring an extra cooler. We decided to use canned beef and fish, so we wouldn't have to worry about keeping the meat cold. And I would pack up all her pills and supplements into plastic bags and containers.

Rana loved camping—she loved waking up in the tent and looking out through the mesh screen at the squirrels. She slept curled up at the foot of our sleeping bags. She loved exploring the woods and going for hikes. Trudy had been camping many times in her day, but she was now almost fourteen years old and had limited mobility, so she stayed home with a pet-sitter. We were camping with Lisa and Joe, and Rana adored the extra attention from other dog lovers. Our advance planning paid off, and we managed her food successfully.

Mike and I had scheduled a vacation to Bar Harbor, Maine, and Acadia National Park for September, a couple of months after the camping trip. We had not planned to bring Rana, but after her diagnosis, I insisted. Fortunately, we had made reservations at a small cottage that allowed dogs. The cottage even included a kitchenette so we could prepare her food.

It had now been five months since Rana's diagnosis and there had been no changes in her behavior. She had already lived longer than the prognosis from her oncologist, and I was relieved, but wary.

Mike's main concern was about Rana's behavior during the car ride. As a puppy, she had suffered from severe carsickness, and used to drool profusely during even short rides. She had outgrown the carsickness, and while she enjoyed car rides, she was always restless and constantly trying to get into the front seat. At around forty-five pounds, she was too big to sit in the driver's lap or paw at the console. Driving with Rana involved endlessly elbowing her to get her to stay in the back. We tried to tire her out before a car ride, taking her to the woods and throwing sticks for her, so she would lie down in the back seat. Unlike Trudy, who felt quite at home in the car, it seemed to take Rana forever to settle. And once she did, even the slight movement of the car changing lanes on the highway could rouse her from an apparently sound sleep and get her moving around again.

We left for Maine a couple of weeks after my agility mishap. The crutches and cane were packed in the car; this would not be the active hiking vacation we had planned, at least for me—Rana would still get to run on the beach. My injured foot lay propped up on a pillow as Mike drove. On our way out of town, we stopped at a store to purchase a dog harness that would attach to a car seat belt for Rana. It fit her securely, and we belted her into the back seat, next to the cooler, pillows, and other vacation supplies. Mike breathed a sigh of relief. Problem solved! We were ready to begin our journey, which would take several hours.

Back on the road, strange noises emanated from the seat behind us as Rana twisted and squirmed, refusing to relax.

"What on earth is she doing back there?" Mike asked.

I turned around. "Ruh-roh."

Somehow, in a matter of minutes, Rana had managed to free herself from both the harness (including the seat belt), and her regular collar. As I looked back, she gave one last shake, kicked off the last of her trappings, and cheerfully launched herself forward to occupy her preferred position between the two front seats, tail wagging. It was reassuring that she was still herself, still earning her middle initial of *T* for Trouble, still making us laugh.

I was working at the clinic after we returned from Maine when Linda, one of the technicians, pulled me aside.

"There's a really nice cat here from the Neady Cats shelter who got neutered today," she said. "I believe he was found in a parking lot. I know you lost your cat a while ago, so I thought you might be in the market for a new one."

I thanked her and said I'd have a look at him. I hadn't been thinking of getting another cat—not yet. However, I knew that sometimes the right animal comes your way even when you aren't expecting it. I remembered a client who had told me the cat I'd come to see was known in their household as the "spare" cat.

"We already had two cats when we found out he needed a home," she explained. "We didn't want another one. But then my father said, 'Well, you can always use a spare cat.' So we kept him." The "spare cat" had become a well-loved family member.

I thought of another client, an elderly woman named Doris who had called me for a home visit to examine her new kitten. The woman's husband had recently died in a car accident, and her daughter had given her the kitten as a gift.

"I didn't want a kitten," Doris declared when I arrived. "But my daughter found this kitten as a stray, and she told me she's a pure-bred ragdoll kitten so she's *really valuable*. So I took her, and now I love my little Sally. I just love her so. She's been such good company since my husband died. And she's worth a *lot* of money, you know!"

At the time, a ragdoll kitten cost somewhere in the range of $1,000 to $2,000. Sometimes more. I could tell Doris was very proud of that.

But I took one look at the kitten and saw immediately that this was not a purebred at all. She was an ordinary domestic longhair, the sort of cat that shelters are full of. I thought about telling Doris that her cat was not valuable, not in the way she meant. It would be wrong to lie to her about her cat's breed. But just as I was about to say something, Doris grabbed my arm. She said, "I'll show you the pictures of the car my husband was driving when he died." The photos were right next to her on the coffee table. I could tell she really wanted to show them to me. "See, can you believe it? No *wonder* he didn't make it."

I realized then what believing in this cat's economic value meant to her. It was a way for this elderly woman to make sense of the horrible thing that had happened, by believing that even if luck had passed over her when it came to her husband's death, she had gotten lucky here, with Sally.

There was no question in my mind that Doris and Sally needed each other. I picked up my pen and Sally's chart. Next to the word BREED, I wrote *Ragdoll.*

When I had a break in appointments, I sought out the cat Linda had recommended. He was a light buff-orange tiger who seemed friendly. I picked him up, and he purred against my hands. I brought him out of the cage and into an empty exam room for a better look. Though clearly an adult cat, he looked quite young, and was happy to get out of the cage. One of his back legs was deformed, and he hopped around, seemingly quite agile despite his disability. I picked him up to inspect the paw more closely. The leg itself was shortened, with only three toes instead of four, and there was a small split, or fissure, going up the middle of the paw. I couldn't tell if he'd been born with the deformity or whether it had resulted from an injury when he was a kitten.

It was the cat's back left paw, I realized. The same paw in which Rana had sustained two broken toes after being run over by a car, causing her to be brought into the clinic where she and I met. The same foot, also, that I had injured in agility class. The Family Boo-Boo Paw. It appeared this cat would fit right in with our household. I brought the orange cat home, and Mike and I named him Marula, after an orange African fruit.

Marula had been home for less than a week when I brought him back to the clinic. Trudy and Rana, used to living with a cat, had accepted him easily, and he was unconcerned with them. We were keeping our new cat, but I wanted to take some X-rays. Something else was wrong with him, I'd concluded, after watching him hop around the house for a few days. He had a funny, crooked gait that I couldn't attribute solely to his shortened back leg. I thought his hip may have been dislocated, an injury not uncommon in cats who have been hit by a car or had another trauma. If this was the case, he would need surgery, but would have a good prognosis afterward, especially if I could keep him from becoming overweight so as not to stress his bones and joints.

At the clinic, I put the X-rays up on the light box viewer. I looked first at the pelvis. It looked fine; the femur bones were both settled nicely in their respective hip sockets. Nothing looked wrong there.

"What's that?" asked Dot, the veterinary assistant who had helped take the X-ray. She pointed to an area of the spine above the pelvis. I raised my eyes up higher and saw what appeared to be two fused vertebrae.

"Wow, I don't know!" I responded. I called the other vets over who were working that day and we looked at the radiographs together, hemming and hawing. We also noticed that Marula seemed to have an abnormal curvature of his spine. We had taken an X-ray of his left rear paw, and he was missing metatarsal bones in that leg, so I now knew he had been born with his funky paw, along with the other defects.

I did some research on my new kitty's X-rays. The malformation was called block vertebrae, I discovered. A veterinary neurologist told me he saw it occasionally and that it could be an incidental finding and did not typically cause pain. I was much relieved. I didn't care if my cat walked funny, as long as he wasn't in pain.

Marula was a perfect pet for a veterinarian, I realized. Anyone who works at a veterinary clinic is likely to adopt animals with "issues"; the assorted pets of veterinary clinic staff are typically some combination of one-eyed, three-legged, partially paralyzed, diabetic, behavior-challenged, and so on. Veterinary and staff pets tend to resemble creatures from the Island of Misfit Toys—the Land of Misfit Pets. One technician, Chris, had a pug named Annie who was paralyzed in the back end. A small dog, Annie was able to get around well enough by dragging herself with her front legs and she was a happy little thing. At the clinic, she hung out with the receptionists behind the front desk. Their favorite comment from surprised clients was "Is she *always* like that?" They longed to respond, "No, on weekends she walks normally!"

In addition to his conversation-starter status (in veterinary circles, at least) from having an unusual medical issue, Marula turned out to have a winning personality. He was incredibly social, materializing promptly whenever visitors arrived, jumping into laps, preening and showing off. He had an easy purr and enjoyed being the life of the party. Living with him, we found, was like living with several cats. He was active and interactive, following us around, playing with Rana, decimating plants, and generally getting into trouble. He was the type of cat who would seem to be sleeping on the sofa one minute, then would suddenly appear in the middle of the room you had just walked into, as though he could teleport. We thought we had mice until we figured out it was Marula getting into the kitchen cabinet and eating bread. He could get in—and out—of the cabinet quickly enough for the door to close behind him, so we did not suspect him until we glimpsed him casually exiting the cabinet one day, licking his lips. Eventually Mike affixed a strong magnet to the cabinet door, and Marula was unable to paw it open.

Due to Marula's extroverted personality, he had several offers of adoption from friends and family members. Mike, typically after cleaning up one of the cat's messes—dirt from a dug-up plant, or pilfered grocery items—liked to grumble about *that cat* being returned in a hurry if anyone did take him. Nonsense, I would say. *That cat* is not going anywhere.

One day when Lisa was visiting, she made what Mike and I considered the consummate remark about our cat. "He really is a great cat," she observed, scratching his orange-striped head after hearing yet another Marula story, "but I'm kind of glad he's not *my* cat."

16

A Good Death

A woman once called me to discuss a euthanasia appointment for her dog. She was not my client, and I had never met her or her dog. She told me about her dog's medical condition and treatment, and we discussed the option of euthanasia. It wasn't quite time yet, she explained, but she was exploring her options in advance.

"He's been a great dog, and he's had a really good life," the woman explained. "I want him to have a good death, too."

I never ended up meeting the woman or her dog, but I'm grateful to her for the way she spoke openly about her pet's death. We don't seem to know how to talk about death, for ourselves or our animal friends. Euthanizing an animal is often termed as "putting down," "putting to sleep," or even, sadly, "got rid of." Veterinarians talk about "making a decision." Our cultural uneasiness regarding euthanasia is reflected in the awkwardness of the language surrounding it. Yet the word *euthanasia* itself comes from the Greek language, and the literal translation is "good death." Even as we dance around the term, people continue to seek out euthanasia for their pets.

For most of us, as much as we dread their loss, we dread their suffering more.

One of the main differences between veterinary and human medicine is having the option of euthanasia for my patient. After so many years of euthanizing animals, and so many conversations about it, it is difficult for me to imagine treating patients *without* the option of euthanasia. It doesn't seem natural, to be forced to wait until someone dies "on their own," the veterinary term for a non-euthanasia death.

Companion animals typically have much shorter life spans than humans. It's common for people to find themselves, either suddenly or inevitably, having to make the heartbreaking decision to end their beloved pet's life. As a veterinarian, I can advise and recommend but not choose. The decision to euthanize always belongs to the owner. My recommendations, however, must be given with great care.

When the topic is euthanasia, medicine becomes art.

Many veterinarians find clients more appreciative about euthanasia than any other service we provide. Perhaps most telling is that I often hear people say, "I wish this was something we could do for people."

Many years ago, I worked with another veterinarian named Johnna, who taught me a valuable lesson. Johnna had a patient, a little dog who had somehow developed a large abscess on the top of his head. Upon treatment of the abscess, some drainage proceeded to drip into one of his eyes, causing an eye ulceration. The unfortunate little dog was quite a sight, with his head covered in drains, sutures, and scabby crusts, earning him the clinic nickname of Frankendog.

Frankendog was hospitalized for a few days to care for his wounds, and the veterinary assistants gave Johnna a hard time. She and I were both new graduates, and the staff was unused to our approach to veterinary medicine, in comparison to the approach of the newly retired owner.

"Why are you keeping that dog alive?" they asked. "It hurts to look at him! Don't you think you should tell his owner to put him to sleep?"

Johnna was not one to mince words. "I don't care what he *looks* like! I know he looks awful. What counts is how he *feels*. He's eating, and once everything heals, he'll be okay again." Eventually, Frankendog did heal, and went home to enjoy the rest of his life. And once the fur on his head grew back, he looked just fine.

Frankendog taught me to look beyond the superficial in assessing quality of life, and to question any preformed assumptions I may have developed.

Quality of life is a slippery thing to define, and the owner is often in a better position to rate the pet's quality of life than the veterinarian; I think of Frankendog and try to make sure I am not being swayed by appearances. Yet I also must guide a client in denial about their pet's condition or their impending loss.

Occasionally, a client will inform me they have consulted an animal communicator and asked them to speak telepathically with their pet regarding the euthanasia decision. At first this confused me. Wasn't it my job to help the client understand how the pet is feeling, whether they are comfortable or suffering, what their quality of life is? Veterinarians are trained to seek signs of discomfort, recognize patterns, and predict how a condition may progress. We observe and examine the patient. With the benefit of experience, we interpret our findings and communicate them to the animal's owner. It's hard for me to understand how a person, no matter how gifted, could tell over the phone or from a photograph what an animal they've never met is thinking and feeling. I try to keep an open mind; perhaps there are people who have such a talent. There are so many things about animals we don't understand. Yet when I see a client who is talking about getting advice from an animal communicator, I typically see a person who is deeply conflicted.

Making a euthanasia decision is never easy. In fact, the best word I've found to describe it is *excruciating*. I do believe it's a blessing to be able to relieve suffering, and I know most clients feel the same way. On the other hand, I've seen many people racked by guilt and an overwhelming sense of responsibility over the decision to end their beloved pet's life. It's a difficult place to inhabit, the space between life and death, all hinging on a judgment many people feel unqualified to make. Yet the animal's human is their next of kin, and, along with their veterinarian, they know their pet better than anyone else.

That fall, about six months after Rana's diagnosis, Trudy started to fail.

My beloved first dog had turned fourteen years old a few months earlier, and she slept most of the time. She could no longer navigate the seven steep stairs to the fenced backyard, so we'd set up a tie-out in the front yard, where there were only two and a half steps.

The tie-out worked well for a while, but eventually she struggled with that, too, as even the two and a half steps became too much for her. I tried a ramp, but she refused to use it. At seventy-five pounds, she was too big for us to pick up easily, and she resented any attempts to help her. At one point, she fell outside, in the rain, and I had to struggle to help her, both of us miserable.

Winter was coming.

Trudy could not hear nor see well, but that didn't concern me, provided she was comfortable. I had put Trudy on pain medication, which she now was unable to function without and could barely function with. I tried acupuncture as much as she would allow, but she didn't like to be touched, or even patted, and retreated into herself.

In New England, we often need to take the weather into account when we consider euthanasia. If Trudy was struggling now, I knew it would only get worse with the snow, ice, and extreme cold temperatures of a Massachusetts winter.

I agonized. I cried. I went back and forth. It was excruciating to live in this limbo of decision-making. It seemed different from what it had been with Daiquiri; he had become sick so quickly that it had felt as though I didn't have a choice. With Trudy, it felt more like a decision that was in my hands: her health was more stable, with one day not much different from the next. Yet I knew that if I waited too long, I risked having to euthanize her as an emergency if she fell and injured herself. Although we try to give our beloved friends the "good death" they deserve, it doesn't always turn out the way we planned. A "not good" death, whether by euthanasia or not, can happen despite our best efforts. As regretful as it might be, the manner of death does not define a life.

I considered Trudy's quality of life. My dog was just existing. She didn't even chew tennis balls anymore or show any interest in fetching, which had been her lifetime passion. Although she was still eating, she was fading away.

It was time, I concluded.

With some clients, I've observed an emphasis on choosing the exact moment to end their pet's life. I've seen people focus on scheduling the procedure not a moment too soon, and not a moment too late. I felt this way about the decision to euthanize Trudy. Amid my emotional anguish, the importance of choosing not just approximately the right time, but *exactly the best moment* to end my beloved pet's life seemed to acquire enormous significance, perhaps because it was the only thing I could control. With the benefit of hindsight, I can recognize that I placed unnecessary additional pressure on myself during a difficult and painful time. Ultimately, I decided to do what I've often advised clients to consider: I chose a day and time when Mike and I would have time to grieve afterward, without having to rush off to work.

I spoke to Alycia, my veterinary school classmate and coworker at Eileen's clinic. While Alycia did not know Trudy well, she had known her since she was a puppy. She agreed to come to my home and euthanize Trudy the day after Christmas.

Part of the veterinary culture is never to call in sick; if we do, it will necessitate the rescheduling of multiple clients. Veterinarians also tend to be perfectionists. We generally do not quit, or stop, until the job is done. There's a push-through mentality for almost everything. On occasions when many people would be sent home for a sick day, most veterinarians will continue to work, provided they remain upright and not at a human hospital.

If one works with other veterinarians, is it possible to ask another veterinarian to perform a euthanasia for you, say, if you are having a bad day? You could, but it rarely happens due to emotional reasons—it is more likely to occur due to a scheduling matter, such as a doctor getting tied up with an emergency or a surgery that took longer than anticipated.

That Christmas Eve, I was working at the clinic, along with Alycia. Because I am Jewish, I didn't mind working so some of the other veterinarians could stay home with their families. Before appointments started, I had a look at the schedule. I noticed my last appointment of the evening was a euthanasia. The clinic had a policy of trying to schedule a euthanasia as the final appointment of a workday. That way grieving clients wouldn't have to sit in a waiting room filled with other clients and we as veterinarians and staff would be able to focus on the euthanasia appointment without worrying about running behind. I groaned inwardly. In a matter of hours, I would be in the same position as the client in the appointment book.

The euthanasia appointment happened to be tasked to me, but it was not a patient I had been seeing. I glanced over at the schedule for Alycia and noticed that her last appointment was not marked as specifically for her. That meant neither client had requested a specific doctor and their appointments had been randomly assigned to whomever had an open slot. It occurred to me that I could ask Alycia to switch with me, so I wouldn't have to perform a euthanasia less than forty-eight hours before my own dog was euthanized.

I pondered the idea for a moment. I had never made such a request before. Could I ask that? Would it be *very* selfish of me? My emotions around grief and loss felt close to the surface, and I decided this aspect of self-care might be okay. I asked Alycia, who agreed, as I would have if another veterinarian had asked me. While it was hard for me to make the request, it felt good to take care of myself, and to realize that it was okay to ask for help.

Christmas came, and then the day after. Trudy did not have to even get up from her dog bed in the living room. I fed her pieces of peanut butter sandwich, her favorite treat, as Alycia gave the tranquilizer injection. After a few moments, her chewing slowed, and she placed her head down. Alycia gave the final injection as I stroked Trudy's beautiful brindle-and-black fur, the fur I would no longer be able to see and touch every day as I had for the past fourteen years.

Trudy rested.

She was an awesome dog, my Trudy, and she'd had an awesome life.

She had a good death, too.

For the next few days after Trudy's death, I woke each morning with the sense that something was terribly wrong, before remembering that my companion of fourteen years was no longer with me. *No, no, no, not that. Not Trudy. Not that.* My belly ached with grief.

I doubted myself, too, experiencing guilt just as I had seen so many clients express both before and after making a euthanasia decision. I have seen people experience these feelings for not recognizing a situation soon enough or for not making the decision at the right time. They feel somehow deficient in their pet's care, as if they didn't love them enough. The fact of their animal's illness, their death, makes some people feel like a failure. They feel lacking. Rather than thinking *if only*, they think, *if only I . . .*

If only I had done this, or seen that, or made the appointment sooner . . .

They blame themselves.

Yet all we can do, as animal caretakers, is to make the best decisions we can with the information we have at the time. And while many people move beyond those feelings, recognizing they are undeserved and unhelpful, others may remain stuck there, forever experiencing potent negative emotions whenever they think of their beloved pet.

Hindsight is twenty-twenty, I reminded myself. It was one of my friend Karen's favorite phrases, and it fits so well in this situation. It is often easy to second-guess yourself after the situation is resolved, with what you now know. I also knew that grief alone was hard enough to bear without the addition of unnecessary guilt.

"Your oupa used to say there is no death without guilt," said my father. I wished I could talk to my grandfather about his experiences, and about why issues surrounding death and dying seem to trigger many people's deepest, most painful guilt responses.

I've even heard people apologize to their pets as I give the euthanasia injection, the words *I'm sorry* merging with *I love you* as though the emotions themselves are intertwined. It breaks my heart to see people suffer unnecessarily during such a painful time. Sometimes I think that the stronger the love, the more people blame themselves. In the vast majority of cases, the intense remorse I've watched so many people experience over decisions surrounding their animal's death has been unwarranted.

Perhaps because of my medical training and experience, I did not feel overwhelmed by guilt and shame regarding Trudy's death. The moments of self-doubt I experienced were temporary; uncertainty was a place I visited briefly but I did not take up permanent residence there. I knew I had done my best in each individual moment, with each individual decision.

When I found myself in the land of self-doubt, guilt, and shame, I discovered a way to pull myself out. I reminded myself of the love I shared with my friend. Then I asked myself, *would Trudy want me to feel this way?*

The answer was always the same: *Of course not.* She loved me, and she knew how much I loved her. She knew my heart. She would not want me to suffer, to dwell in a place of pain. I followed her love out of the land of guilt, as her love set me free.

On the third day after Trudy's death, it snowed. And I felt something other than grief and guilt.

Relief.

Trudy didn't have to physically struggle through this day. It still felt awful that she was gone, and I still missed her terribly, but it also felt right.

Both Trudy and Daiquiri were now gone. I had lost my first adult family. My head was a jumble of our time together and our adventures, as our stories together had come to a close. I drew comfort from my new family, Mike, Rana, and Marula.

17

The Red Dot in Winter

Rana loved winter as she loved all other seasons: fully. She loved to play in the snow, and one of our favorite winter games was to shine a laser pointer through the windows of the back porch into the backyard at night. The Red Dot, as we called it, showed up well in the snow. We could make Rana run in any direction we wanted. She would charge along, mouth open, leaping like a gazelle after the Red Dot. Mike and I took turns getting Rana to run in circles or figure eights and change direction. When we turned off the laser, she would stop and put her head down, staring at the precise spot in the snow where the laser pointer had been. When we turned it back on, she pounced on it with joy. It was great fun to watch her run in all directions, getting her exercise while we remained cozy and warm inside.

The only problem was getting Rana to come back in. Using the laser pointer to lead her indoors did not work. Long after we turned off the Red Dot, she'd still be outside, staring at the snow, convinced it was about to reappear so she could give chase. Once I even tried tossing some tortellini from that night's supper outside onto the top step to try to entice her back in. Of course, she just ate them and ran off.

As Rana was doing well, I began to have moments of peace. I still ordered her herbs and supplements in one-month supplies, not daring to order more, but I didn't worry as much about each month being her last.

I stayed in touch with Steve Marsden, emailing him about once a month with an update. Steve's responses were always generous and thoughtful. Many times, he responded with a suggestion for something else to add to her list of supplements. Steve's philosophy of holistic cancer treatment did not involve a search for a miracle cure. Rather, treatment consisted of individualized support for the patient through diet, lifestyle, supplements, and herbs, while also utilizing treatments that had been found to have some anti-cancer activity. At times, he would recommend I contact other holistic veterinarians, to hear their thoughts. These wise colleagues in other states and as far away as Australia were gracious and helpful as well. I felt honored to have the help of so many pioneers in the field of holistic veterinary medicine to advise me with Rana's care.

I also took Rana back to see Dr. LeVan a couple of times, bringing homemade chocolate chip cookies to show my appreciation for her care. Rana was happy to visit her friends at the veterinary dental office, and they were always glad to see her. Laura was concerned about Rana's gum tissue/tumor, which protruded out of her mouth. To prevent it from drying out, she recommended applying Aquaphor, a Vaseline-like ointment, to the surface daily. She also recommended an oral rinse.

One day, I came downstairs and said to Mike, "I don't think anyone will ever love me the way Rana does." Later, it occurred to me those words may have been hurtful to him. I would have been upset if he had said them to me. I emailed him at work to apologize for being thoughtless. *Don't worry*, he responded, *I'm not upset.*

I continued going to yoga class, where my teacher Ann often talked about the concept of "comfortable discomfort": having a part of the body relax while another area works hard on a pose. She also stressed the importance of continuing to breathe throughout the pose. It helped me realize that I could feel sad about Rana's diagnosis while still enjoying each day with her.

Sometimes, I would hug Rana, much as I had done that time on the love seat. *Not today*, I would whisper to myself, thinking of how happy she was. *Not today.* It became a mantra for these moments of peace. I still didn't know what the future would bring or what tomorrow would look like, but at that moment, we were together, and we were okay.

Rana was now five years old. I didn't know her exact birthday, only that she was about four or five months old when I first saw her on May 1, 2000. I had always thought of her birthday as January 1, 2000; I imagined her birth occurring at the precise moment of the beginning of a new millennium. A special birthday. Perhaps she had a perfectly ordinary birthday, like December 15 or January 3. She was still special to me. And she had made it to five.

Rana lived each day to the fullest, just as she always had. Her appetite was tremendous. In fact, I had increased her food, because she was getting a little bit thin, and had some muscle wasting on her forehead. This cancer cachexia is common in both human and animal cancer patients; it is the reason many cancer patients lose weight. Rana was now happily eating substantial amounts of food and, just as happily, generating substantial piles of poop. Her coat shone from the canned salmon in her diet; Mike and I joked about what they must think of me at our local Trader Joe's, where every week I nearly bought out their supply of canned salmon.

As well as Rana kept doing, her tumor stubbornly insisted on growing. It was hard not to notice it, there at the very front of her body; it preceded her into a room. It was the first thing I saw when I opened my eyes in the morning, as Rana loved to stand on the bed and stare at me as I woke up, her tumor mere inches from my face. By now the mass had grown far out of her mouth, and her enlarged gum area was protruding. She appeared to have buck teeth.

One person who saw her thought she was holding a tennis ball in her mouth. "No, that's just her mouth," I had to explain. As well as growing forward, the mass now extended upward to her nasal cavity and backward toward her blue eye. Other than the deformity reminding me of her limited life span, I didn't care what she looked like. That came as a relief, because when she was first diagnosed, I didn't think I could bear to see her disfigured. Only when I looked at photographs of her was I amazed by the transformation. Otherwise, she was still Rana. Rana T., because Trouble was her middle name.

I had my eye on a large blood vessel in the front of Rana's mouth. It was quite near the surface and ominous looking. I began grinding all of Rana's medication with a mortar and pestle, not wanting anything sharp to rub against the large blood vessel.

Rana showed no signs of being in pain, but I worried, nonetheless. I consulted an oncologist; which pain medication should I start Rana on? I didn't want to do anything that could contribute to bleeding. Other than a lot of sneezing, Rana was acting fine. The sneezing didn't seem to bother her at all, but I always worried it would trigger a nosebleed (it never did). The oncologist recommended a pain medication and I started her on it. I didn't notice any difference in her behavior, but I didn't want to take a chance that she was having pain I was not addressing.

Before Rana, I had treated many animals with cancer, including my own cat. Daiquiri's tumors, however, were well hidden from my view. Some cancers were external, like Rana's, with changes easily seen and noted. Others were buried deep inside the body, difficult to monitor, an invisible, silent time bomb. Would it be easier to forget about a tumor if I didn't have to look at it all the time? Would that make the reality any less painful? Perhaps I would worry more if I couldn't monitor the tumor's growth as easily.

I realized that, before Rana's diagnosis, despite all the patients with cancer I had treated over the years, I had never fully comprehended just how individual each tumor is. Out of a full three dimensions, in which direction would a particular tumor grow? What paths would the blood vessels, so haphazard in their unsanctioned growth, forge in their uncharted exploration? In one hundred, even one thousand animals with the same tumor type, it was possible that no two tumors would grow in the exact same way.

I felt a peculiar relationship with Rana's tumor. On the one hand, the tumor was a part of her, literally inseparable, the surgeon had told me. Those cells were *her* cells, 100 percent Rana. How could I not love them, too? On the other hand, that tumor would take her away from me too soon, cheating her of the life she deserved. Sometimes I felt that the Cancer—capital C—was another being that lived in the house with us; an uninvited, ill-mannered houseguest who stubbornly refused to leave. At times, it felt as though the Cancer gloated, waiting for me to remember its presence if, for a few moments, I managed to forget.

I considered the popular "fight" analogy regarding cancer. People always talked about "fighting" cancer. I didn't want to picture a battle going on in my beloved dog's body. I wanted Rana and her cancer to coexist peacefully. I wanted them to agree to disagree, for as long as possible. As a doctor, I couldn't help but wonder if medicine—both human and veterinary—could benefit from this type of approach. The mechanisms of cancer development and growth, I knew, were the same in humans and animals. I longed to talk this over with Oupa and discover his thoughts on the subject.

As I grappled with what was going on in my dog's body, Rana herself remained unconcerned. She lost a couple of teeth as the tumor grew. I saved them in a medicine vial, her precious DNA. She still chased her tail daily and delighted in the home-cooked food, and she swam after ducks until it became too cold to swim.

Rana loved to stand at the back door, which had a window almost to the floor, and gaze out into the backyard. It was her form of television. She would look first in one direction, then turn her head to look the other way. Her tail would remain down, relaxed, until she noticed something interesting, when it would slowly rise to curl over her back. If she noticed something suddenly, such as another animal, her tail would rise swiftly, and her head would arch backward as she did what we referred to as her "Dino bark," because she sounded like Dino from the Flintstones. *Ruh ruh ruh ruh roooo!!* I could watch her for hours.

"You are obsessed with that dog," Mike would comment, shaking his head, and I would smile in agreement.

One night, unable to sleep, I got out of bed and crept downstairs. I wanted a miracle, so I searched for one online. I had done this already, on many nights, after Rana was first diagnosed. By this point, I knew all there was to know about maxillary fibrosarcomas in dogs. But what if I had missed something? What if there was something new, something Steve hadn't told me about?

I scoured websites boasting of miracle cures for canine cancer. I read compelling testimonials that I knew may not be true. I knew these companies were selling products, and anyone could create an appealing website targeting people like me. But I was vulnerable; I wanted to believe.

Some of the products were supplements I was familiar with, but many contained ingredients that the holistic veterinarians I knew, leaders of the field, had discounted as unhelpful. Some could even be harmful. Just as in human medicine, there are many fads about the latest miracle cure for pets.

I clicked and read, clicked and read. Eventually, I checked out academic sites, too. There was a study going on, I learned, a clinical trial taking place at a veterinary school a thousand miles away. A new medication. No, it wasn't for Rana's type of cancer, but the write-up mentioned the protocol might one day be applicable to her type of cancer. We could fly there, I decided, I would bring her there, I could call in the morning and see about the study . . . finally, I stopped myself.

There would be no miracle cure. There would be no flying off to participate in a study. My beloved dog had already gone an entire year since her diagnosis. She was happy, every single day. I already had a miracle. It just wasn't going to last forever.

I trudged off to bed.

Not long afterward, I was at the clinic examining a dog with cancer. Sam, a friendly terrier mix, had a large tumor on his side. His owner had elected to forgo surgery when the cancer was first diagnosed several months earlier, due to financial reasons. Now the tumor had grown and was too large to remove. Sam's owner was interested in holistic treatment, and after examining Sam and having a lengthy discussion with his owner, I recommended a diet and some supplements.

"Last night," Sam's owner confided, "I couldn't sleep. I'm so upset about Sam. I ended up going online, and I ordered something, a dog cancer medicine, some kind of supplement. It was seventy-five dollars. I know it probably won't make any difference. But there were so many dogs on the website who had done so well . . ." She looked at me, tears in her eyes.

"He's just such a good dog," she added.

I've been there, I told her, as I explained about Rana. Up in the night, searching for a miracle, reading testimonials with an open mind and a heavy heart. I have been there, myself.

"He's a really good dog," I agreed as I patted Sam's soft fur at the end of the appointment. "A really good dog."

18

Veterinarians in Crisis

In today's fast-moving news cycle, emotions in general are often compressed. We are inundated with stories and not encouraged to dwell on any one narrative for long. Last week's headlines now seem dated and obsolete, hence the phrase *that was so five minutes ago*. When a loss occurs, we are encouraged to treat it the same way, even though each grief experience follows its own timeline and is more likely to ebb and flow over a lifetime than resolve during a matter of days or weeks.

And people sometimes underestimate the importance of their relationship with their pet to their life's story. The connection of a human with a dog, a cat, or other animal can be one of the deepest bonds of a person's life. Many are emotionally shattered when faced with a difficult diagnosis or the loss of a beloved pet. And yet, this intense grief may go unseen and unrecognized, and therefore, unsupported.

There is a name for this experience: disenfranchised grief. *Dis-*

enfranchise means to deprive, and *disenfranchised grief* is the experience of feeling that your grief is not recognized by your community. It can be an isolating experience.

Some people are lucky, like me. My friends, family, and coworkers respect my relationship with my pets either because they feel similarly themselves or because they know I am a veterinarian and can therefore be excused for my strange behavior. But many grieving pet owners are subjected to thoughtless comments from those around them:

Why are you still upset over your cat?
Wasn't that a long time ago?
Just get another one the same color.

Even those who are sympathetic may not comprehend the depth of the relationship. Veterinarians and their staff may be the only ones to understand how a grieving client feels.

Veterinarians are commonly confronted with not only animals in crisis but people in crisis. We deal with the emotional fallout of an emergency as well as the injured or ill pet; the shock of the owner whose pet slips out the door and is suddenly hit by a car; the person coming to terms with the imminent death of their pet after a slow decline. That animal may be the being they are closer to than anyone else in the world.

Despite having no training in the field of social work, veterinarians increasingly find ourselves acting as therapists as we help clients work through difficult decisions and the grieving process. We may suggest grief counseling, but many will not seek it out; some feel a stigma for being so upset over "just an animal."

Fortunately, a new field called veterinary social work has emerged. The field seeks to address the needs of both pet owners and veterinary staff. The mere existence of this type of social work is both validation for veterinarians and a testament to the strength of the human-animal bond. Many veterinary schools now have a veterinary social worker on staff, to offer support for clients, as well as support for veterinarians, staff, and veterinary students.

However, most clinics do not employ a social worker. Much like my grandfather was, we are alone in the room when we give the news nobody wants to hear or to speak.

Many people become emotional when their pet's life is at stake. I often find it difficult not to get misty-eyed when people are crying, especially if I know them well. I don't consider this a bad thing; I think most people appreciate it. The sound of a person crying in the same room with me is not something I can easily tune out, nor do I want to. Men's tears especially move me, as I know they are so often suppressed. There appears to be something about our beloved pets that lowers the barrier to tears, and I have seen many men cry at the death of their animal.

I have noticed that when men do cry, they may do so awkwardly, clumsily, clearly unaccustomed to the process. Some men's tears appear to leak out without their permission from a deeply buried internal spring, reminding me of the scene from the movie *The Wizard of Oz*, in which the Tin Man—the character who did not believe he had a heart—cries as he says goodbye to Dorothy.

"I've never seen him this upset," wives and girlfriends have confided to me. Men's tears, so rare in our constrained male culture of manning up, seem almost sacred.

Part of the downside of being empathetic about the human-animal bond is the difficulty with controlling and regulating said empathy. I feel strongly for people in the heartbreaking situation of letting go of their animal friends. However, my empathy must be well controlled so I can perform my job and maintain objectivity. If I'm not careful, my own feelings could expand and take over my consciousness. So I hug my empathy to myself. I also can't allow my own painful memories and experiences of loss to surface. I must remain in doctor mode; I cannot put myself in the place of the client. If I did, I would be reliving some of the most painful moments of my own life, over and over again.

If my subconscious has a choice between acting professional and showing emotion, I've discovered it will always err on the side of being professional. Sometimes I feel such a tight clamp on my emotions that I am unable to tear up, even if it would be appropriate. These experiences can be the most difficult for me, and these are the times I am likely to feel numb afterward. I have "manned up," my emotions tamped down and suppressed. For hours or even days afterward, I may feel a peculiar detachment.

Writing a sympathy card to a client can also become an emotional task, even—or especially—after writing hundreds of cards. I try to make each card special, as I know that for some people, my card may be the only physical expression of sympathy they will receive. I choose cards with writing that expresses my sentiments well because despite years of practice, there are still days when I stare blankly at a card and can think of nothing more to add than my name.

Veterinarians are so involved in helping others with their narratives that they often neglect their own, and failure to separate from the stories of clients and patients can lead to burnout and compassion fatigue.

I would love for someone to invent something called an empathometer, a kind of empathy calculator and regulator. Wouldn't it be nice if there were meters and dials that could be set beforehand and if the device came with a manual? *Euthanasia*, I could type in. The device would then present me with a list of questions based on several variables. Clinic visit or house call? How many family members will be present? How long have you known the client(s)? The pet? The external device, which would sync to my internal empath controller, would then supply recommendations. Tears, misty eyes, or nothing? In front of the client(s)? In front of staff? While writing a sympathy card? Or in the car on the way home? For one visit, I could dial down my empathy to, say, a three, and for another one, up to an eight (only for my own pets would a ten be possible). The device would regulate my emotions for me, keeping me in the narrow window of acceptable emotion to be able to do my job and not repress any sadness.

After the procedure, I would input more information into the empathometer. Did I see a man cry? Did the procedure go smoothly? Did I cry? The device would then spit out my risk for compassion fatigue from the preceding event, along with recommendations: *Risk is 5.5; you may not sleep well tonight. Recommend stopping on way home for pint of Ben & Jerry's, call friend, exercise, meditate.* Or: *You need a good stiff drink.*

When I explained my idea to Mike, he came up with something even better. "How about a device you could wear, that would calculate your cumulative exposure to compassion fatigue situations, the way those badges you wear to take X-rays monitor radiation exposure? It could even measure your heart rate, like one of those wearable fitness devices."

"That would be great!" I responded. "Then everyone at the clinic could wear one! The receptionists, technicians, assistants . . . they all could use one."

"And it could let you know," Mike continued, "when you need to take a break."

Some years ago, my internal empathometer communicated to me how hard it was becoming to euthanize pets belonging to close friends and family members. The issue was not solely a matter of maintaining objectivity, because while I may be fond of the animal, the pet is not my own beloved household member. The main difficulty lies in how well I know the person, and how much I care about them, as well as their relationship with their beloved pet.

With clients, I can facilitate some of the most painful moments a person can face by maintaining an emotional boundary. When the client is also a loved one, the boundary becomes far more difficult for me to distinguish. If I have visited a home socially, as a friend or a family member and not just as a veterinarian, there is a different relationship. As personal as the suffering of a long-term client may be, the anguish of a loved one is even harder to bear. When I must battle to suppress my empathy to perform my professional job in such circumstances, the emotional strain becomes enormous.

Certainly, it is something I could do, and something I did for many years. Then I realized that although it may make the lives of all my loved ones easier if I were to be the person to euthanize their pets in their homes at the appointed time, the thought of doing so felt as though it would take years off my life. So I implemented a policy of not being the house-call veterinarian to euthanize the pets of my close friends and family. I will still be your veterinarian, I told my loved ones; I'll still take care of your pets, I'll field your phone calls, texts, and emails at all hours (because as every veterinarian knows, there is no such thing as being off duty when a family member or a friend is concerned about their pet), I'll advise you and be there for you in all other ways. But in this one way, I decided, just this one way, I would take care of myself first.

The issue of boundaries is one many veterinarians struggle with, for good reason. In addition to compassion fatigue, occupational burnout is common among veterinarians. Veterinary medicine is the type of job where you leave when the work is done, not at a certain hour. Emergencies might arrive at any hour throughout the day, wreaking havoc with a schedule of client appointments and surgeries. Clients may arrive late or bring an extra pet, and the care of sick animals can be incredibly time-consuming. Some clients expect veterinarians to give services for free "because you people love animals" (I've often wondered at how that line of reasoning is used so often for veterinarians, but not at the supermarket or pet store). Clients complain about prices even as many veterinarians struggle to pay their own bills. My own car has over one hundred thousand miles on it, as do many of my colleagues'. Some clients have unreasonable expectations regarding their veterinarian's availability during nights, weekends, and days off, even though most of us already work some combination of evenings and weekends to accommodate our clients' schedules. And there are the aforementioned all-hours messaging from family and friends. Sometimes it feels as though I am working all the time.

If my schedule happens to involve a social occasion, such as a barbecue or a wedding, and I admit to the person next to me that I am a veterinarian, I know I will likely be talking about work. While I don't mind viewing pictures of a stranger's pets on their phone, I am more often subjected to a long and detailed history of their (or their parent's or friend's) living or deceased pet's medical crises. I may try to extricate myself, but that is hard to do politely if the person has become emotional. If I am asked a medical question, and Mike is with me, I have begun to have him attempt to answer, as he has witnessed these scenarios so often. For a nonmedical person who is on the squeamish side (other than gutting fish he's caught), he does well, and then at least I get to talk to my husband a bit. Is it me, I have wondered, or do people with other careers have this problem? Would people discuss their leaky pipes or last year's blocked toilet if I were a plumber, or pull off their socks if I were a podiatrist? Perhaps the empathometer should be able to calculate risk for burnout as well as compassion fatigue.

A few years ago, I was visiting a therapist to discuss something unrelated to work. One day as I came into her office, something occurred to me.

"You know, while I'm here, is it okay if, uh . . . if I talk about something to do with work?" I asked hesitantly. "There's a sick dog I've been treating, and . . . well . . ." I faltered.

"Of course," she responded.

It had never occurred to me to talk about work stress with a therapist. I had created my work life to be a good fit for me. I had an awesome career I had worked extremely hard for and which I enjoyed, even though I didn't earn much money. And dealing with euthanasia and end-of-life issues was a part of my job, it was what I did, and it was okay, even when it was hard. I was strong, and I could do my job. I had put up the boundary about not euthanizing pets belonging to friends and family members to protect myself, which was a relief. The sick animals I saw on a regular basis, I talked about a little bit to Eileen or others at work. Sure, there was a case with a house-call client I was involved in at the moment, a situation about a dog with cancer that was keeping me up at night, yet I had never considered seeking *therapy* over it.

But something besides my own stress was troubling me on that day.

I had discovered that the veterinary profession has a high suicide rate. Multiple studies show estimates placing veterinarians at about four times the risk of suicide as the general population, significantly higher than for physicians or dentists.[§]

Suicide? Veterinarians?

"Are you sure you don't mean veterans?" asked my husband when I told him.

Suddenly the news was all over the veterinary press. A well-known veterinary specialist in California had recently died in a

---

[§]   If you are experiencing mental health–related distress or are worried about a loved one who may need crisis support, call or text 988 to reach the Suicide & Crisis Lifeline. For more resources, see page 293.

high-profile suicide, and another veterinarian had died by suicide in New York after enduring a cyberbullying campaign against her. Every veterinary journal and magazine had articles about suicide prevention, as well as articles trying to figure out why the trend might be occurring. What factors could be contributing? Veterinarians are high achievers, sensitive, perfectionists, the articles said; we work long hours, we are people pleasers, we suffer from compassion fatigue and burnout. We have a high debt-to-income ratio. Clients condemn us on social media, which can lead to intense stress and financial difficulties. We have access to euthanasia drugs, and maybe vets are less afraid of death . . .

I had never been suicidal, but I was spooked. I *had* suffered from depression, which was also seen in much higher numbers among veterinarians than in the general population. I had known one veterinarian who had died by suicide; it was the veterinarian who had given me the bad news about Rana after her MRI, the news that had dashed my hopes of a cure for her. At the time, I had thought of only myself and my husband and our beloved dog; but of course, the news must have been hard for her to deliver to me. I'd also heard rumors about other veterinarians I'd known.

What was going on in my profession?

Lisa now worked with international refugees seeking asylum, so she was no stranger to vicarious trauma. Once, she had asked me about the stress of performing euthanasia. "It's not the hardest thing I do," I'd told her firmly. "The hardest thing for me is giving people bad news." As I spoke, I had sensed a barrier deep inside myself, a resistance to talking about work stress, even with someone I was as close to as Lisa.

And it was true that delivering bad news was a source of stress. For me, the most difficult time to deliver bad news is when a client has no idea their beloved pet has a life-threatening illness. It is the client who believes their animal is temporarily a bit under the weather, perhaps resulting from an infection or some other treatable condition; the client who enters the clinic fully anticipating they will leave with some medication, and everything will be fine.

As I speak to the client and examine my patient, my suspicions will grow until they form a hard knot in my abdomen. Depending on the condition of the animal, and how well it fits a pattern, I might even be apprehensive from the very beginning of the appointment.

I remember the first time I ever felt that way, during my first year in practice. I remember where I was standing in the room, and the look of affection on the woman's face as she reached over to stroke the head of her middle-aged black Lab, while she and I discussed the dog's recent fatigue and lack of appetite. She was concerned, but not worried. As she spoke, my fingers found the lymph nodes on the dog's neck. They were several times their normal size, and I knew instantly the dog likely had lymphoma (he did). I knew as soon as I touched the dog's throat that I was going to have to utter words that would change this woman's emotions from love and concern to bitter sadness.

So it was difficult, delivering bad news. How did that compare with euthanasia, though?

I had to peel through several layers of mental barriers to consider this question. Denial: it's not hard. Stoicism: I can deal with it, no matter how hard. Repression: there are some things we don't talk about; we just don't go there. *Do not disturb*, the barrier clearly states. I considered some terms we rarely, if ever, discuss in veterinary medicine: *moral stress* and *vicarious trauma*. One article stated that veterinarians face ethical dilemmas three to five times per week, leading to moral stress, such as when a client requests euthanasia although the animal could be treated or when a client refuses to euthanize a suffering pet. And vicarious trauma is considered to result from empathic engagement with a traumatized client.

I'd been denying the negative effects of veterinary practice for so long that it came as a shock to realize others could be affected, too. I had thought it was just me who struggled.

———

I was working at the clinic one evening, seeing acupuncture appointments, when I realized there were a total of four euthanasia appointments—an unusually high number—scheduled for the evening. I told the other veterinarian who was working that I would take at least one of the appointments. The staff decided I could take the appointment for Misty.

Misty was a cat who, though not very old, was in complete kidney failure. She had been hospitalized at the clinic for several days. The entire family had been in to say their goodbyes and had spent an hour visiting with her in a private room. I watched as the female client left with three school-aged children in a cloud of sniffles and crumpled tissues. Her husband remained behind to be present for the euthanasia.

The visiting room at the clinic was a more relaxing space than a typical exam room, furnished with comfortable seating but no table. Misty's owner had chosen to settle on the floor, with Misty on a blanket. Alone in the room with Misty and her owner, I sat down on the floor with them. While speaking softly to the unconscious, sedated cat, I slid the needle into the vein, which promptly collapsed. Misty's leg was swollen with fluid due to the kidney failure, compromising the integrity of the vein. I explained to the owner I was going to have to use his cat's other front leg to give the injection (as with people, some animals will have better veins on one limb than another). Fortunately, Misty would not mind; she was completely sedated from the initial injection.

The man was crying softly as he said "I love you" to Misty. I knew he had just spent an hour in the room with his family saying goodbye to her. This man wanted the euthanasia to be over. When I explained to him that I was going to have to use the other leg, he moaned. I turned the cat around, ever so gently, and repeated the procedure to give the injection. This leg was even worse than the first; although I placed the needle directly into the tiny vein, it collapsed, and the solution refused to flow. The syringe containing the solution was now clouded with blood, and when I told the man I needed to briefly leave the room to get more, I felt as though I were performing emotional torture on him.

"No," he groaned.

As I went out to get more euthanasia solution, a technician named Hope was folding laundry and asked if she could help. I hesitated. My first response was no, as due to my house-call work I am used to performing euthanasia procedures alone with the client, but then I reconsidered. Perhaps some moral support would be a good idea. Hope could also hold off the vein on the back leg. "Yes, thank you," I responded, grateful for the offer.

Back in the room, Hope and I positioned Misty for a back-leg injection. I was able to visualize and inject her back-leg vein, yet it too collapsed after I began the injection. Misty had some of the toughest veins to inject I had ever seen. The man moaned again; his pain seemed excruciating. My patient, the cat, was not suffering, but the man in front of me was. I had explained about the swelling, but he was beyond explanations.

I considered the next step, which, other than attempting to inject the cat's remaining back leg, would be to inject the euthanasia solution directly into the heart. This is a technique utilized by veterinarians occasionally, in such situations, when we are unable to access a vein. It's not difficult to perform on an anesthetized animal, but it's hard to describe the procedure without it sounding brutal and primitive. I couldn't imagine explaining to the heartbroken man in front of me what I needed to do next.

Then, a shocking idea occurred to me. Although the cat was sedated and had just stopped breathing, the heart was likely still beating; however, I could lie to the owner and tell him his cat had died. Then, as soon as he left, I could give the injection into the heart.

I couldn't believe this had come into my head. I had never lied about a patient, had never even considered it. I had certainly never told anyone their pet was deceased when it wasn't. But this man appeared to be in severe emotional distress. While I felt a moral obligation to not contribute further to his anguish if it could be avoided, I also felt morally obligated not to lie. With effort, I pushed the thought away. I would not compromise my integrity, even to spare someone great pain.

As I sat there on the floor with the grief-stricken man and the anesthetized cat with the swollen limbs, about to discuss the injection into the heart, I came to a realization.

Misty had died. I felt it; I *knew*. There had been a sea change in the room. I had not been aware of the exact moment of her death, but I was now aware her presence was gone. Misty must have absorbed enough euthanasia solution from the tiny amounts I had been able to inject (in addition to the tranquilizer) to cause her death. I put my stethoscope on and listened for a heartbeat. Sure enough, there was none. Misty was gone. I felt relief that Misty's owner had been spared from another injection for his beloved cat.

Every veterinarian has experienced difficult euthanasia procedures; they are etched into the fibers of our beings. To be sure, most euthanasia procedures go smoothly. Yet there are many aspects that can be difficult for those watching. An animal may vocalize and cry out, appearing to a distraught owner to be in pain, even if they are exhibiting only a reflex or a reaction to the anesthesia. Occasionally an animal will experience a seizure or spasms; a respiratory pattern termed agonal breathing is common at the end of life, when an animal is unconscious, and may appear as though the animal is gasping for breath. Some animals, like Misty, have veins that are difficult to access, necessitating multiple attempts and injections. Intravenous catheters, if present, can fail. Other animals will take in a surprising amount of euthanasia solution while stubbornly remaining alive.

Fortunately, these occurrences are uncommon, and clients often remain unaware of these possibilities. Only the veterinarians and veterinary staff, striving to create the best possible experience for both owner and animal, are conscious of what can go wrong.

When I saw Hope at the clinic a few days later, she brought up the experience right away. "That euthanasia appointment was *so hard!*" she exclaimed. "I was really upset afterwards. That poor man, he was *so* sad."

As we spoke about the encounter, I realized I was surprised to hear Hope had been upset after the experience.

Both Hope and I had witnessed a man in the grip of profound sadness and grief. Yet I had been in the room from the beginning. I had overseen the situation and I had performed the euthanasia. I had gone as far as to consider lying to a client. If Hope was upset after her experience, didn't it make sense that I would be upset, too, after mine? And I *had* been upset afterward: professionally, by my failure to inject the cat successfully and create a better experience for the client; emotionally, by the man's obvious suffering; and ethically, by my impulse to lie to the client.

If I had compassion for Hope's experience, I wondered, should I also have compassion for my own?

The day I talked to my therapist about work, I spoke about a dog with cancer I'd been treating in the home. My client was extremely attached to the dog, and I felt so bad for her that I described myself as being "enmeshed" with the situation. The therapist shook her head as she explained that it was not healthy to take on the emotions of my clients. I needed better emotional boundaries.

Veterinarians may act like we are superhuman—in fact, we pride ourselves on it. It's a part of our identity: the stoicism, the persistence, the perfectionism. But perhaps that's not always a good thing, I realized. Maybe we need to show compassion for ourselves, as well as for our patients, clients, and coworkers. We can't afford not to.

19

Rana in Summer

One day, I was walking Rana in the park when I ran into a group of people walking their dogs, and one of them called out my name. I recognized one of my house-call clients, Kate, and realized she was with her dog Molly. While I often recognized a dog before I recognized their owner, this dog was different. Molly was incredibly fearful of anything veterinary related, even at her home. Whenever I saw Molly, she was muzzled and shivering with fear, every muscle taut. Out for a walk in the park, she looked completely different: relaxed and happy. As Kate and I chatted, Molly ventured over and sniffed me, and her entire body language instantly changed. She tensed and backed away from me, hackles prickling. It was as though she had suddenly realized the devil was in her midst.

I was not surprised that Molly knew me by smell. Humans often underestimate animals; many people assume they don't remember people or animals they haven't seen in some time. Yet although they live mindfully in the moment it doesn't mean they don't have memories. When someone asks me, "Do you *really* think my dog/ cat remembers who you are?" I like to tell a story about a cat named Marlowe.

Marlowe was a cat I'd seen only once before, on a house call, for a checkup and vaccines. A year later, Marlowe's owner Ruth called, and we scheduled an appointment.

When I arrived, Ruth had already placed Marlowe in the bathroom as requested. I sat down in Ruth's kitchen and asked her how he was doing, and we chatted about Marlowe's health as I drew up the vaccine and made some notes in his chart. When I was ready, Ruth went into the bathroom to get Marlowe. She was good at holding him, so she planned to bring him to the kitchen table for me to examine.

Ruth was in the bathroom for a couple of minutes. Then she called out, "He's gone!"

Alarmed, I ran into the bathroom. At that moment, Ruth spotted Marlowe. The poor kitty had wedged himself in between the washing machine and the wall, in a desperate attempt to hide. Ruth and I were stunned.

"Is he usually shy when people come over?" I asked Ruth as we removed her cat from his hiding spot.

"No," she replied, shaking her head, "not at all. In fact, I've been having some construction done, and we've had contractors in and out of the house. He's been annoyed, but he's *never* hidden like this before."

Marlowe had recognized my voice, my smell, or both, from my single visit one year earlier. The previous appointment had been uneventful, although it had apparently left a strong mark on Marlowe's memory. I'll admit I was disappointed, but by then I was used to the fact that not all my patients were happy to see me. A couple of people have even told me their cats have run off to hide after hearing my voice on the answering machine.

Rana was different from Molly and Marlowe; she was happy to go anywhere and meet anyone. When I occasionally brought her to the clinic with me, she enjoyed seeing my coworkers and the other animals. One day I brought her for moral support when I went in for a noontime staff meeting; Eileen and I had arranged that I would give a short presentation about acupuncture that day.

My coworkers and I gathered in the doctor's office, a large room filled with desks where we wrote up our charts and made phone calls. Chairs were dragged in from exam rooms and the waiting area, a closed sign was placed on the door, and the telephones were turned over to the answering service. Some people who, like me, were not working that day, arrived with children or pets in tow. Smaller animals waking up from anesthesia were held in laps, and the animals who lived at the hospital, such as Earl the orange cat, were in attendance, as well those who regularly came into work with their owners.

When it was time for me to speak, Eileen offered to hold Rana. I passed her Rana's leash, but my dog was not content to sit on the floor. She clambered into Eileen's lap, all forty-five pounds of her. Spying Eileen's coffee mug on her desk, Rana stretched her neck out and helped herself to a few laps of coffee. We all laughed at her antics, and my anxiety about the presentation vanished. My dog could make herself at home anywhere.

I had thought the previous summer would be Rana's last, but the season had rolled around again, and she was still here. Rana ran and played, and even chewed on soft dog toys with her misshapen mouth. She swam in the lake again, chasing ducks, trying to fly.

We brought Rana camping, and unlike the previous summer, when Mike and I had needed to create a complex plan regarding the coordination of her diet, this time we packed everything up automatically, without even a conversation. Her food preparations had become routine.

We also brought her on a family camping trip with Mike's brother and sisters and their children. Unfortunately, it rained most of the time, and we were confined to our tents, unable to have much of a campfire. In between rain showers, we took Rana for a walk around the campground. As we returned to the campsite, Rana spotted a package of cupcakes brought to celebrate a family birthday. Our niece Sandhya, holding Rana's leash, was unprepared for the sudden surge of energy from our opportunistic dog. Towing Sandhya behind her, Rana dove at the cupcakes, mouth open, emerging from the package with orange frosting and rainbow sprinkles covering her face. We laughed until we cried. Rana's cupcake adventure ended up being the highlight of the camping trip.

Back at home, despite her deformity, Rana chased her tail daily. It began when she caught sight of the extremity. She stared at it as though the crooked tail was taunting her, daring her to chase it. Her eyes narrowed as she accepted the challenge. Next followed tight spins and galloping paws as she spun around and around at lightning speed, her own tail remaining maddeningly out of reach. Eventually, she'd catch the crooked end of her tail in her mouth and walk in slow circles, clearly dizzy. Finally, she'd flop down, exhausted, or come over to me for some attention. Both she and I never tired of the tail-chasing game.

After a swim in the lake one day, Rana's tumor began to bleed. The blood was coming from the nasty-looking superficial blood vessel I'd been watching for months, the one in the very front of her mouth. It bled and bled, like a nosebleed. Fortunately, Mike was home, and together we managed to stop the bleeding. My squeamish husband did not say a word as we cleaned up the mess. Rana did not appear to be in any pain, but she was unusually quiet after the bleeding episode.

Frantic, I emailed Steve. Did this mean it was time to make a decision? Steve told me about a wonderful Chinese herb used to stop bleeding. He recommended giving it to Rana orally as a pill, as well as using it topically as a powder to stop the bleeding. Reluctantly, I decided it would be best if Rana stopped swimming, since it seemed to make her more likely to bleed. I could tell her time was getting closer, but we seemed to have a reprieve with the Chinese herbs.

Mike and I were trying to get pregnant. We both felt that caring for Rana had been good practice for caring for a child. I had also thought Rana would be the perfect dog for a child to grow up with. I felt certain she would keep me company when I was up at all hours with a baby. She would curl at my feet, as she loved to do, while I rocked the baby in the still of night. It was a scene I could picture so well, so clearly. But I realized it was not going to happen.

Around that time, I did a house call for a client named Larry who had lost a young dog, a beautiful Great Dane named Sampson, to severe heart disease the previous year. We talked about how hard it was to lose a beloved pet so young. Larry had done everything medically possible for his dog, consulting specialists and spending thousands of dollars, despite Sampson's poor prognosis. Much like myself, he had left no stone unturned.

That day, Larry told me how angry he was at the breeder. She should have known there was heart disease in the line of dogs, he declared, eyes flashing. We both knew that Great Danes are prone to a certain type of heart disease, which can be hereditary. How could they have bred those dogs, he asked me bitterly, knowing there was the possibility of heart disease in their line?

I recoiled from his anger in surprise. Unsure how to respond, I tried to turn the conversation back to what a wonderful dog Sampson had been and how friendly Alfie, his other dog, was. But later, I thought about Larry's words again. Larry's situation had been so like my own. Yet I did not have a focus for anger. I didn't have anyone to blame for Rana's cancer. My emotions had ranged from shock and disbelief to despair. Perhaps my lack of anger was due to my medical background. We know there can be a hereditary element to cancer, as certain breeds are more prone to develop it. But just as in humans, researchers believe the cause is multifactorial—that many factors can contribute to a cancer diagnosis—and much of the time, the veterinary or medical profession has no idea why an individual gets cancer.

What if I felt anger? I wondered, would it be any easier for me, if I had someone to blame for Rana's abbreviated life? Recalling Larry's flashing eyes, I didn't think so. I was having a hard enough time coping with the current situation. Would the anger take the place of some of the pain and sorrow I felt, or would it exist in addition to it? If I felt someone—or something—was responsible, I concluded, any anger I experienced would feel like an additional burden. I felt grateful that anger was not something I had to face.

One day, as summer drew to a close, Mike found me in the kitchen.

"We need to talk," he said.

I closed my eyes. I did not want to have this conversation.

I knew what he was going to say. Mike thought it was time. He thought it was Time.

I did not.

Rana's tumor was enormous, the size of an orange. I had added more pain medicines to her lineup of medications, preferring to treat something that wasn't there rather than risk her suffering untreated pain. There had been an infection inside her mouth, and I needed to keep her on antibiotics or the infection would return.

If I had examined Rana as a patient and the owner decided it was time for euthanasia, I would have agreed without hesitation.

She was clearly on what I consider the spectrum of time for which euthanasia was an acceptable choice.

Yet she danced and played, ate and ran. She looked like a happy little manatee. Once, when we were out for a walk, a couple of high school–aged girls had walked by me and Rana, heading in the other direction. I noticed them staring at Rana as they approached. After they passed us, they burst into spontaneous giggles, undoubtedly at the funny-looking dog they had seen. I felt like turning around and yelling, "She has cancer! She's the best dog in the world! How *dare* you laugh at her!" Instead, I looked down at my dog. Rana's mouth was open, her tongue hanging out. Her eyes were bright and her ears pricked forward as she scanned the horizon for squirrels. She was having a great time. She was oblivious to the mean girls; only I was upset.

Another time, Mike and I walked her to the park down the street, passing by an enormous mastiff tied up in a yard. We had seen the dog before, and he was easily three times Rana's size. That day, his owner was outside with him. As the mastiff's owner caught sight of Rana's mouth, with her protruding teeth, we heard him nervously call his dog over to him. "Zeus, Zeus, c'mere! Yikes, check out the *teeth* on that dog!" Mike and I almost doubled over with laughter thinking about Zeus's owner perceiving our little Rana as a threat to his giant dog.

Mike and I sat down on the sofa in the living room together.

I knew it was common for pet owners to disagree about the precise time for euthanasia of their animal. The difficulty of decision-making is even harder when couples or family members differ in their opinions.

"Look at her face," he began. "How much worse can it get?"

"I know, I know," I responded. "But she's so happy! She's eating! She's playing!"

Mike knew Rana was more my dog, and it was ultimately my decision. He was not going to insist, but he wanted to say his piece. I knew I had to listen; I needed to respect his opinion, and I did not want to be blinded by my love for my dog. As impossible as it was to be objective, I knew I had to consider Rana, primarily, in my decision. It didn't matter whether I was ready or not if it was her time, if she was suffering.

Often, I and other veterinarians encourage clients to look for a sign, either an obvious clue such as not eating or something less obvious, what we often call "a look in their eyes," that they are ready. Trudy had exhibited such a look, and I had seen it in the eyes of many patients. Rana, in the prime of her life, was less likely to exhibit such a look. But I still expected to see something that would let me know it was time.

"I know it's soon," I said to Mike, struggling to control my emotions. "I know that. I know she doesn't have long. But I just don't think it's *right now.*"

Mike nodded slowly in agreement.

"Hey," I said suddenly, looking around, "where is she, anyway?" Typically, if Mike and I were in a room, Rana was there, too. She was nowhere to be seen, and the house was suspiciously quiet.

That dog was up to something.

I got up and went into the kitchen, where we had a gate set up to prevent Rana from getting into the pantry. The gate was elevated off the floor by several inches, enough to allow Marula to walk underneath, but not Rana. Cat food and kitty litter were in the pantry, and if the gate was open, our dog loved to sneak in and eat the cat food or raid the kitty litter.

The topic of our conversation was currently flattened to the floor, with her head and shoulders on the wrong side of the gate, her front legs splayed out to the sides, and her back legs stretched out behind her. She had somehow managed to grab the bowl of cat food with her deformed mouth and was slowly dragging it back under the gate in a type of limbo dance/backward army crawl. She was licking the cat food from the bowl as she reversed her flattened body, and began licking faster as I approached, realizing she had been discovered.

I smiled broadly, my peace of mind temporarily restored. I had never been so happy to catch my mischievous dog in the act. Rana had given me a sign, a good sign, one that reinforced my sense that we had a little more time together.

"If she's still getting into trouble, it's not time yet," I told Mike firmly.

Mike smiled and shook his head. "What a goof," he said, looking at Rana.

20

Rana

When I see a person deep in grief over the loss of their pet, I encourage them to tell their animal's story by creating an obituary. Many people have thanked me for the suggestion, and some have shared their writings with me.

While stories can provide information and help us remember, they can also help us heal.

Of course, animals cannot write their own stories, but we can write the stories of our lives with them. The first time I heard of a pet obituary was many years ago, after a friend who worked at a bookstore asked me to participate in a pet loss panel. During the panel, a middle-aged woman sat in the front row and spoke about her little dog who had died earlier that year, and how difficult she was finding it to accept the loss. Then she mentioned writing an obituary for her dog. "An *obituary?*" I responded, wide-eyed. It was a light-bulb moment for me. The woman explained that a therapist she was seeing had recommended it to her. The process had helped her, she said. I told her I loved the idea and was going to recommend it to my clients.

I admit to a history of newspaper obituary reading. I like obituaries because they tell a story, and I love stories. It's also a way to learn about people in my community. If I read about a stranger, sometimes I'll wonder: Did I ever stand behind this woman, who so enjoyed cooking lasagna for her family, at the supermarket? Or I'll note, *isn't that sweet, they listed his dogs as part of the grieving family left behind.* Many obituaries follow a set format and are somewhat formal and impersonal, but sometimes there are true gems buried in them, glimpses into a person's life story as seen from the end.

Perhaps that is why I latched on to the idea of writing obituaries for our beloved pets after they die. I don't mean publishing something in the newspaper, although I wouldn't be opposed. I'm talking about writing something from the heart, to help the heart heal.

It doesn't have to be formal; it is more a matter of putting pen to paper (or fingers to keyboard) while focusing on the history of a beloved pet's life. An obituary may describe a pet's personality, quirks, and adventures. It is a way of telling their story and the story of your life together.

Many years ago, I euthanized an enormous dog who was not my patient. The dog was unable to get up at all when I arrived at the house. The owner shared a few details of his dog's life. "He's even been to California," the man revealed, adding, "*I've* never been to California." When my friend Dina's cat Tigger was near the end of his life, she coaxed him to eat by pureeing shrimp in a blender, ignoring her children's pleas for the pre-ground delicacy. Tigger had been a part of Dina's family since before her children were born, and she was happy to spoil him with shrimp smoothies.

Our connections with our animal friends can be profound. Pets are often the first things we see in the morning and the last ones we see at night. There's an immediacy, an intimacy to our bond with them. After her dog's sudden death, a client confided to me, "I've had family members die and I haven't felt this bad." When we live with someone, they become family; even, in a sense, a next of kin. Consider a relative who lives in another state and with whom you may have a complicated relationship, and then consider a beloved pet whom you see daily. You may not think of the human family member every day, whereas you think of and interact with your pet multiple times per day.

Pets inhabit our homes in a manner difficult to explain. On a day when our dogs were at the groomers, my husband commented how noticeable their absence seemed. "Even though they would probably just be sleeping right now," he said, "the house feels so different without them here. Why is that?" The breaths, the heartbeats of the animals who live with us, contribute to the very heart and soul of a home. And they can linger long after an animal has gone.

During my time with Lisa and Joe in Mexico, we visited a small town in the mountains to observe the celebration of Day of the Dead. We saw an altar with dozens of candles by the roadside on the way to the cemetery. At the graveyard itself, high on a hill, the sky was cloudy, and mist swirled around the gravestones. Yet the town-wide festival had a cheerful air. Whole families gathered with picnic baskets. Children played while adults chatted and scrubbed the stones with sponges and soapy water. They also tidied the area and arranged flowers. Each gravesite appeared unique, with distinct features and decorations, like a neighborhood with a variety of houses. The visitors seemed to be enjoying themselves, and no one appeared to be in a hurry. It was clearly not just an annual cleaning that was happening at the cemetery that day; it was a time to maintain connections with lost loved ones.

Those connections, even after a person or animal has died, are something I think of often. Just because our loved ones are no longer with us does not mean that the love is gone. They are still a part of our lives and our stories.

When I have written obituaries for my own pets, it is a way of grieving, of memorializing them, of sharing their story with others and keeping it close to me. It is a way of telling my story as well, the story of my relationship, my love, and my loss.

Obituaries can help us heal.

As September stretched into October, Rana had more bleeding episodes. She did not seem affected by them, but it was stressful for me and Mike, trying to get the bleeding to stop, cleaning up the mess, wondering if it would happen again.

Knowing her time was drawing near, Lisa and Joe invited us to spend a weekend at Joe's parents' cottage on a lake in the Berkshires. Lisa and Joe left their animals at home so Rana would be the only dog. She enjoyed the attention and long walks. One afternoon, Joe and Mike took the canoe out on the lake while Lisa and I sat on the shore. As the sky darkened into evening, the air chilled, and Rana, who didn't have much body fat, began to shiver. Lisa removed her own flannel shirt from the back of her chair and put it over Rana, carefully fitting her front paws into the sleeves and fastening the buttons. Rana stopped her shivering, and both she and I were warmed by our friend's love.

On the way home from the Berkshires, we stopped at a nearby apple orchard. Rana was in the back of Lisa and Joe's station wagon, separated by a dog gate from the rest of the car. As we came back to the car carrying apples and cider, Rana greeted us from the front seat. Once again, our Houdini of a dog had wiggled her way out of an enclosure.

A couple of weeks after we returned, I noticed Rana's back paw reach over to try to scratch her face, something I hadn't seen her do since the tumor had grown. Before I could stop her, she proceeded to give a good hard scratch—then yelped in pain and stopped. I comforted her immediately, and she appeared to shake it off, watching out the window for squirrels a few moments later, but I was deeply troubled.

That night, I heard Rana up in the night, licking. Just licking. She was uncomfortable, restless, there at the foot of the bed. This had never happened before. I got out of bed and brought her into the little half bathroom next to the bedroom, the place where my kitty Daiquiri had retired to when he was dying. There, we didn't have to worry about waking Mike, and Rana settled down in my lap as I sat on the floor with her and soothed her. I could tell she was uncomfortable. I spoke to her and patted her, stroking her soft ears, telling her how wonderful she was and how much I loved her, as I reached the conclusion I had been dreading for so long. Eventually, Rana settled and seemed comfortable.

Her discomfort had been my sign, I knew. It was Time.

The next day, I told Mike, who nodded in resignation. Then I called Lauren, another of the veterinarians at the clinic. I asked her if she would come to my house in a couple of days to euthanize Rana, and she agreed. Everyone at the clinic knew what was going on with my dog and had been following her progress. I felt bad asking Lauren to help me, as I knew it would be difficult for her. I hadn't wanted to euthanize the pets of family and friends, and Lauren was a close coworker of many years. But at the time, there was no one else euthanizing animals at home except for me. With Trudy, I had wanted her to die at home because she was anxious at the clinic. Rana would have been fine at the clinic; I wanted her to die at home so Mike and I could mourn in private.

After the bad night, Rana seemed to be herself again, untroubled and carefree. Yet I was not going to change my mind. It had been so hard to see her in pain, and I didn't want it to happen again, as I knew it would. I considered prescribing her a morphine patch, but I worried it would be difficult for me to monitor her comfort level. While I dreaded our separation, I didn't want to keep her alive if she was in pain.

Lisa suggested we get together the night before Rana died and volunteered to come over. That evening, Lisa, Mike, and I took Rana for a walk to the park she loved, a place where she had spent many happy hours sniffing, running, greeting other people and dogs, chasing squirrels, and fetching sticks. She saw several squirrels during the walk, and Lisa took lots of pictures. Back at home, we had pizza and wine for dinner. We were all amazed that Rana had retained the ability to catch food tossed to her, even with her enlarged mouth. She must have eaten most of the cheese from the pizza, catching it in midair. The conversation was all about Rana, and she was patted and spoiled even more than usual. It was about as good of a last night as it possibly could have been.

Later, Lisa told me she had taken not only pictures that night but also videos. She eventually worked with her brother to turn them into a slideshow, set to the music of Jack Johnson, showing Rana darting after a squirrel, catching pizza cheese, and being patted and loved by all of us.

The following morning, Lauren arrived. Mike went upstairs to the bedroom because he did not want to be present. Lauren gave Rana the tranquilizer injection. It took Rana a few minutes longer than most animals to feel the effects, likely because the rest of her was in such good shape—other than her tumor, she was in excellent health. While we gave the tranquilizer a few moments to calm her, Rana somehow managed to get away from us and ran upstairs, searching for Mike. One last Houdini escape. Finally, we got her back downstairs and onto the couch, where the sedative took effect.

Lauren injected the euthanasia solution into her vein, and Rana was gone.

I sobbed. I couldn't believe she was dead. I didn't want her body to leave—I wished I could have kept just one of her soft ears. I caressed her and talked to her until I realized I wasn't being fair to Lauren. Eventually, Mike, Lauren, and I brought her out to Lauren's car. I ran to get some flowers to go with her and then gave her soft forehead one last kiss. When Lauren drove away, the pain seemed unbearable. It felt as though my skin was peeling off my body. I was bereft.

Later that day, Mike and I, both red-eyed and bleary, went for a walk. We went to the Audubon Society trails, a place we didn't normally go to because no dogs were allowed, and we always took Rana with us when we walked in the woods. On that day, I didn't want to see any other dogs, not yet. As we hiked the forest trails, I thought about the many times Rana had run through the woods, and Mike and I later discussed how we both could feel a part of her with us during that walk. I resolved to always remember her and to never minimize the bond we had shared. It was special, I told myself. I will never pretend otherwise. I know she wasn't my child, and she wasn't human. But she loved me so much, and I loved her so much. And she should have been able to stay. She should have grown old, as my other animals had been able to do.

When we got home from the walk, I didn't know what to do with myself. I walked around the house aimlessly, from room to room, feeling that even the house would never be the same.

Finally, I sat down to write an obituary for Rana. I wrote about her life; how full it was and how she both gave and received a lifetime's worth of love. I wrote about how, when I first saw her, I fell instantly in love and felt like the Grinch when his heart grew three sizes that day. I wrote about how joyous she was, how mischievous, and how Mike called her the "empathy dog" because she always knew when one of us was upset. I wrote about how much we would miss her.

I wrote a story of love and sorrow, family and loss. Connection that transcends species, space, and time.

The story of Rana.

Our love for Rana, our caring for her together, had deepened our connection with each other as well as with our dog. The love we shared, I knew, would continue even after her death; it was as strong as silk, as soft as her ears, as real as my breath. It would outlast us all.

21

The Rana-Colored Thread

My pain in the days after Rana's death was immense. I had thought I might feel better, just a little, after she was gone. I'd imagined that perhaps the end of the waiting would be a relief. Yes, the worrying was over. When, Where, and How was now known. But it was not enough. I missed her constantly, violently. The feeling of peace that eventually came to me after Daiquiri and Trudy died refused to appear. She had been so young, in her prime, while they had lived long, happy lives, and were blessed to grow old. Rana's loss felt unnatural. And despite all the death and illness I had seen in my work, I was not desensitized. If anything, I was more sensitized, having empathized with so many people about their losses over the years. Now it was my turn, and it hurt so much, so deeply.

I moved through the days in a fog, going through the motions but not feeling present. The emptiness in the house was palpable.

One good thing about being a veterinarian is that friends and family assume you are crazy about your animals. Everyone who knew me was aware of my love for Rana. Although not everyone understood my feelings, I received a lot of compassion, which helped, because every day—every hour—without my dog felt like a challenge. Once I sent out Rana's obituary via email, sympathy cards began to arrive in the mail, and I read them over and over.

I created a temporary shrine with photos of Rana, sympathy cards, and her collar. Looking around the house, I was surprised to realize there were some of her things I seemed to need around me, while other things were difficult to have near me. The sofa cover we had on our old sofa fell into the latter category. Rana had napped and snuggled on that sofa cover, but it had also been where she died, and I couldn't bear to look at it anymore, not for another minute. The feeling seemed random, and irrational, but I didn't stop to analyze it. I removed the offending sofa cover and bundled it up to give away.

Something that seemed illogical in the other direction was a tiny drop of dried blood on the hardwood floor in the living room, left over from one of Rana's bleeding episodes. It happened to be near a knot of wood where it blended in and was easy to overlook, yet once I noticed it, it seemed important for it to remain there. It brought me a peculiar feeling of comfort. I never mentioned it to anyone; certainly Mike would have cleaned it had he noticed it. It was a little piece of Rana hidden in the house that only I knew about, and it remained there until we moved.

Unable to sleep, I found myself up in the night once again, creeping downstairs to my office, this time not looking for a miracle online but for solace.

Pet loss, I typed into the browser, *grief dog died*.

I was amazed at the number of pet loss websites that appeared. Apparently I was not alone. Of course, I knew that already, having seen so many grieving pet owners over the course of my career. But I tended to see and talk to them more before their pet's death and directly afterward than in the days that followed.

On the computer, alone in my home office, I surfed through websites, finding pictures, stories, poems, even a video of a woman singing a song about her beloved dog. One website had created a weekly virtual candle-lighting ceremony, with participants from all over the world.

There were many, many people who felt as deeply as I did over a pet's death.

One day I called Mike at work, frustrated. "This stupid health insurance website," I complained. "It's having me jump through all these hoops to find an authorized provider. I put in your social security number, since you hold the insurance, but now it wants something else. It says—for an additional security question, it's asking for the name of your first dog. What was your dog's name, when you were a kid? Was it Buffy? Muffy? Something like that, right?"

There was silence on the line, and for a moment I thought Mike was no longer there, that we had lost the connection. Then I heard him clear his throat.

"Rana," he said simply. "The answer is Rana. She was my first dog."

I knew Mike had bonded to Rana, but maybe I had underestimated how important she'd been to him. Like me, he loved her, cared for her, and made sacrifices for her. It felt as though she had made the two of us a family. Discovering this hidden window into Mike's relationship with Rana confirmed to me just how special she'd been, to win over my dog-phobic husband and earn his love, and how deep his grief was for her.

Some days later, I was in the shower when it occurred to me that I was feeling a tiny bit better. My emotional pain was not as all-encompassing as it had been, I realized. The intensity was lessening. However, instead of feeling pleased by this insight, I was unexpectedly overcome with sadness and longing. There, enclosed in a beige-colored plexiglass shower stall, I doubled over.

The ache I felt was not for Rana herself, but for my own grief. At that moment, it was the pain itself I missed. I had felt closer to Rana in the deep, intense anguish of my immediate grief. It was a poor substitute for Rana herself, but it was all I had. I didn't know what to do without it. I didn't *want* to move forward, I concluded. Each day brought me further and further from Rana's physical presence, her touch, her smell, her sweet self. Soon, I worried, those memories would start to fade. The pain was as close to Rana as I could get, and I wanted to stay there, to remain in my cocoon of sorrow.

Slowly, I pulled myself together. I tried to breathe normally. I got out of the shower, dried off, dressed. I recalled that after Daiquiri died, I had thought about all the millions of cats in the world, all the cats who looked like him, all the other gray tiger cats out there. How could none of those millions of cats be Daiquiri? Our neighbors across the street had a dog who looked sort of like Rana—at least when viewed from across the street. Mike and I referred to the dog as "the Rana clone." Could there be another Rana clone somewhere? I knew I had seen her after she had died, had put her into the back of Lauren's car, but could she be somewhere else?

That was the night I dreamed of the Rana-Colored Thread. The dream came to me when it was almost morning, during the in-between time, when I was not fully asleep, yet not awake. I have always had vivid dreams, especially in the time between wake and sleep, in the early morning. Sometimes I'll partially wake and begin thinking about the dream, then fall back asleep and continue it, inserting a half-awake thought. At these times my dreams often seem incredibly real. This time, as I woke, my perception of reality was altered, and I believed fully in what I had experienced. I woke up repeating to myself, "Rana-Colored Thread, Rana-Colored Thread."

This is what I wrote that morning:

> *In my dream, there is a thread connected to me, leaving me and disappearing, as if into a cloud. The thread is attached to Rana. I know this with certainty. I know that we are attached to one another, because I feel the connection through the thread. I feel it even though I cannot see her, and I don't know where she is. The thread is the color of Rana, which is the color of sunlight and fresh baked bread; it is as soft as the fur on her ears. It is as real as our love.*

Because I knew this in my dream-wake state, I did not question. What thread? Where does it attach to me exactly? At what point does it disappear? It didn't matter. I just knew that it was there, and I was deeply comforted. It helped me with the hardest question, which is this: Where, exactly, is Rana now? Rather than answer this question for me, my new knowledge made the answer seem less important.

I couldn't have Rana anymore, but I would always have the connection to her, wherever she was, a connecting thread made of love. Rana-colored love.

22

Stories of Medicine

One day, my father discovered a folder with some old papers of his father's, writings no one had known about, tucked away in an old briefcase my grandmother had kept. Oupa had died more than twenty years earlier, and I was thrilled to find this hidden link to his thoughts. *Musings of a Medical Minnow*, read the cover page. Reverently I touched the thin papers, reminiscent of those long-ago aerograms. They were in perfect condition, as though they had just been written. For years I had longed to speak to Oupa about the similarities in our work; here was an unexpected window into his life as a doctor. I read about some of his cases, his interest in psychiatry, and his thoughts about medical practice.

> *In the old days, many a person found comfort in discussing her problems with her family doctor, who was often of real assistance, who listened to her story, and who put things in their proper perspective. Her backache was no more than a mild lumbago—no slipped disc in those days—and*

meanwhile, the real reason for her visit to the doctor was mentioned, and dealt with, almost in parentheses.

Yes, I thought, *this*. Our details may have been different, but I knew exactly what he meant. The woman who called me because her old dog was vomiting but whose real question was "How will I know when it's time?" The confession of a man grappling with misplaced guilt who felt bad about how he had treated his beloved pet, wanting to know if something he did, or failed to do, had caused his cat's cancer. The problems were *in parentheses*.

When I was young, I used to wrinkle my nose when my father asked me if I'd consider studying human medicine rather than veterinary medicine. I had not yet heard the common joke in the veterinary world, "Veterinary medicine . . . *because people are gross!*" I wouldn't realize until I was in practice how much of veterinary medicine involved working with people and how I needed to communicate with my clients to provide the best possible care for my patients.

I always hoped to be a good doctor. But how is a good doctor defined? Is it one who solves a nagging, persistent problem? Who sutures neatly if surgery is required? The one with the good reputation at the good hospital? Who graduated from the good medical or veterinary school?

Or is it about more than science, more than medicine? Certainly, skills and knowledge are required. But perhaps a good doctor is one who looks at you, makes eye contact, and *sees* you; who listens; who knows what is important to you as an individual. The doctor who problem-solves with you in partnership. The type of doctor who tries to identify—and address—the issues hiding in parentheses as well as those clearly defined.

To keep a good balance between the scientific and the human—the interplay—this is what makes a doctor what he is, Oupa had written.

He knew that the practice of medicine was as much about connection as disease. Like my grandfather, I believe I can be more effective if I understand my patients and clients as individuals.

But even in my grandfather's day, the general practitioner was becoming obsolete. Several years ago, I scheduled an appointment with my primary care physician because I'd been feeling unusually tired. At the doctor's office, a nurse took my temperature and blood pressure, then left me alone in the exam room. It was the middle of the day, and I had worked that morning but eaten little breakfast and no lunch in anticipation of a fasted blood sample, so I felt even more tired than usual.

After a long wait, my physician entered the room and sat across from me. She asked me some questions (Was I depressed? Any changes at home?), then left with a promise to perform some blood tests to check my thyroid and see if I was anemic. I dressed and went to the lab area to wait for my blood draw.

Only on the drive home did I realize that my doctor had not touched me at all, not even once.

What would Oupa think? I wondered, as I also considered that I personally would never conduct an examination that way. The only reason I would not touch a patient would be to avoid putting myself in physical danger if an animal was actively trying to harm me. Had the doctor been unusually busy that day? Veterinarians are known for being so busy at the clinic that we often skip lunch and even limit trips to the bathroom. I knew what it was like to be on a tight schedule. But to not lay hands on my patient? That I could not justify.

I don't generally make a fuss; I'm more likely to eat a restaurant item I didn't order than send it back. But this issue seemed too important to ignore. With my grandfather in mind, I called my insurance company and asked to be transferred to another primary care provider. It turned out to be a wise decision. Whether I was pegged as a needy patient or whether it was pure luck, I was placed with a wonderful physician, a doctor like my grandfather. From the very beginning, she made eye contact with me, wanting to know me as an individual, not a problem to be solved.

In his book *Being Mortal*, physician Atul Gawande describes how years ago, most humans lived in reasonable health until an illness or an injury occurred, which often caused their death. With the benefits of modern medicine, it is now possible to recover, fully or partially, from numerous medical problems. Many issues that were once fatal are now able to be either cured or managed on a long-term basis. This is true for veterinary medicine as well.

There has also been an important cultural shift: dogs and cats have gone from living outdoors to sharing our living rooms and bedrooms, and our relationships with them have changed. Fifty years ago, if a cat developed a heart problem, he would have simply lived with it until he died from it, with no one the wiser. The cat would not have visited a specialist who would perform an echocardiogram and prescribe medication to improve the heart's function, a common scenario these days. Veterinary care has come a long way, and so has our willingness to seek it out.

The advent of modern veterinary medicine has increased the number of interactions many pet owners have with their veterinarian and may have even increased the depth of the bond people share with their pet. If you are monitoring your animal friend's health on a regular basis, giving him medication and following up with your veterinarian, you are putting more effort and energy into your pet's well-being, and thus your relationship with him. You may have nursed your dog through an episode of pancreatitis, chronic allergies, or the time she ate two entire boxes of chocolates (that was Trudy). There may have been visits to the emergency clinic for vomiting or coughing, and to a specialist for a chronic problem. The commitment to our animals, the caring for them, strengthens the feeling of them being family. It also strengthens the relationship with the doctor who cares for them, and who has perhaps cared for the last pet and will care for the next one, too.

I first met Dawn when she brought her dog, Henry, to see me at the clinic. Dawn always came to the clinic with her friend and her friend's beagle, George. While the dogs were the same breed, they couldn't have been more different. Whereas George was a typical beagle—howling with indignation at every vaccine, wriggling constantly, and struggling through the whole exam—Henry was the perfect gentleman, calm and serene, even holding his paws up politely for a nail trim. When I commented on this, Dawn told me he'd been her rock through many changes in her life. I could see this immediately, how his steadiness was something she wanted to hold on to.

Less than a year later, Henry was diagnosed with cancer. Dawn was devastated. Henry had been her stabilizing influence all these years, and his decline sent her into a tailspin. Dawn brought him to an oncologist, but the cancer was aggressive and Henry went downhill quickly. When the time came for me to euthanize him, I went to her home. Afterward, Dawn collapsed in my arms. I grieved the loss of him, too. But I also knew this was the moment when I needed to be her rock.

A few months later, Dawn called me with excitement in her voice. I was surprised to hear from her as we hadn't spoken since Henry had passed. Dawn told me she'd heard from Henry's breeder. A litter of beagles had been born that was distantly related to Henry. However, this litter of puppies was special. They all had a rare neurological birth defect which caused them to walk as though they were dizzy. Dawn had fallen in love with one of the puppies and decided to adopt him.

Fred was the happiest little puppy I'd ever seen. He couldn't go two steps without falling over. But he didn't mind this one bit. Neither did Dawn. For someone who had admired her previous dog for being steady, it struck me as ironic that she had fallen in love with a new dog who couldn't walk a line. But then we need different things from our relationships at different times in our lives. We can need an animal who's "steady" only to discover we need its opposite as well.

Dawn moved to New York City but continued to have me as her veterinarian for a couple of years, bringing Fred with her when she came to visit her mother. I loved seeing Fred and hearing Dawn's stories about his adventures walking with a city dog walker. But although we enjoyed seeing each other, Dawn and I reluctantly agreed that it made sense for her to change to a local veterinarian.

Sitting around Dick and Claire's kitchen table one day, I listened to them reminisce about all the pets they'd had over the course of their lives. They talked about the first dog they'd had together, all the way through the pets I had known and treated. It was a way to mark the passage of time, through the animals that have accompanied us through our lives. I loved to listen to their stories. Occasionally, a veterinary student would call me and ask to spend a week with me as an elective. I always brought the student to meet Dick and Claire. Dick loved to show off the tricks he'd taught his cat, and Claire could have Arnell the pig sit for a cookie. "Tell the story about the gas company," I'd say, and Claire, eyes twinkling, would recall the day the local gas company was working on their street. One worker had knocked on their door and requested access to their home. As the man entered their dim front hallway, he spotted Arnell. "What kind of a *dog* is *that*?" he had exclaimed. Thus followed a procession of gas company employees entering their home for a view of this city- and home-dwelling pig.

One day my father, trying to emphasize that an event had oc-

curred many years ago, finally exclaimed, "That was *two dogs* ago!"
That's how we chart our lives, through stories of the family members, human and otherwise, who accompany us through our days.

The stories I loved most were those that showed how animals can fill empty places in our lives that humans are unable to occupy, and how closely our lives are intertwined.

I began seeing a dog belonging to a client I knew, Harold. Several years earlier, I had acupunctured Harold's previous dog, Sierra, a lovely Doberman he always referred to as "Sierra the Good Dog." Sierra the Good Dog suffered from a condition called Wobblers syndrome, a neurological disease common in Dobermans and Great Danes. Sierra had to be carried in for her first appointment, but she responded well to acupuncture. Although she never had a normal gait, she was able to walk without falling or crashing into walls.

Now Harold had come to see me with his aging boxer, Charles, who had just been diagnosed with cancer. Charles was as sweet as his predecessor. Harold, however, was distraught. We sat down together in an exam room to discuss Charles's diagnosis and treatment. Harold was worried about the surgery his dog would need, and I reassured him that with the type of cancer Charles had been diagnosed with he was likely to do well. Harold told me that he himself had been treated for cancer two years earlier.

Suddenly, Harold changed the subject.

"Four years ago," he said with some difficulty, "my son died in Afghanistan. I was going to end it all," he continued, both hands on Charles's fur, "and this dog . . . *this dog* . . . got me through it."

Charles had saved his owner's life, by his very presence.

Fortunately, Charles's condition was treatable. We scheduled surgery to remove the tumor, and follow-up care including acupuncture. Charles went through his surgery with flying colors, and enjoyed his acupuncture treatments, often falling asleep during the sessions.

Many of my patients are geriatric dogs and cats and require extra care, and I see how people adapt their homes to maintain their beloved pet's comfort. The amount of attention an older animal needs may increase gradually, so people don't always realize how much they have worked their daily lives around their pet's unique needs. Some kitchens sport paths of throw rugs to give older dogs more traction on a slippery floor. Older or sick pets may need medication administered multiple times per day or insulin to treat diabetes. Some give their older cats subcutaneous (under the skin) fluids at home to help failing kidneys. Older animals may be up in the night with cognitive dysfunction (dementia), disrupting people's sleep. I've seen more than a few clients abandon their own beds to sleep next to a pet who is unable to climb stairs.

My client Joanne was caring for her dog, Jade, a yellow Lab with terminal cancer. Joanne told me she had nursed both her parents through hospice care. Now she was doing it for Jade. Home acupuncture treatments had sent Jade into remission, which was thrilling. However, now the cancer had returned and was growing larger. We knew it was simply a matter of time before she became uncomfortable.

"She looks for me, and she gets upset if she can't see me," Joanne confided one day when I arrived. "I try to shower when she's sleeping."

One of my clinic clients, Jane, whose dog Betty's arthritis I was treating with acupuncture, had an unusual way to get Betty to shake paws.

"I say, 'Do we have a deal?'" Jane explained. "It's part of something longer I've said to her since she was little."

Naturally, my assistant Michelle and I wanted to hear the whole agreement, and it brought tears to our eyes. The bargain Jane had struck with Betty was this:

"I'll always come home to you.
There will always be food.
And you always come when I call.
Do we have a deal?"

The longer I'm in practice, the more connections I have with my clients; I may remember not only my patient as a young animal but also the client's previous pet. When I see an older patient, I may have followed her through multiple medical issues over several years. When a long-term client's dog was diagnosed with a life-threatening illness, I felt even worse remembering how she had lost her previous dog to cancer at a young age. Each appointment, each conversation, fits into a larger story, an ongoing narrative not only of my patient but of my human client and their lives together.

I've always loved to read, though I used to consider it a guilty pleasure; something I enjoyed but which offered no wider benefit. That changed when I read about a human medical approach called narrative medicine, which involves viewing the patient (and caretaker) in the context of their larger story to better understand and communicate with them. Patients and caretakers can also benefit from narrative medicine, as the concept extends to the patient's own story, and their narrative as an individual. When I take a history from a client, I'm seeking some kind of framework; information about my patients seemed like random bits of data until I assembled them into a story. And *that's* why I don't like drop-offs, when I'm faced with an animal without a caretaker, because it's harder to understand the situation unless I already know the person and the animal well. The narrative model fit well with Oupa's writings, and both our practice styles could be considered narrative medicine.

I may come up with a different treatment plan for a rarely seen barn cat compared with an indoor cat who sleeps on the owner's bed, and I'll need to work with the client to figure out what's effective. A limping dog may need to be confined until a sprain heals, and a vomiting cat may need different food. How will the client medicate the patient, monitor them, and restrict their environment? What that looks like for an individual animal can vary tremendously. Only by considering a wide-angle view of the patient's life will I have the best chance of a successful outcome.

I wondered whether narrative medicine could offer veterinarians a pathway back to my grandfather's style of medicine. Perhaps it could help practitioners view our patients in a full three dimensions, rather than as flattened two-dimensional representatives of a disease or the 10:00 a.m. appointment in Room 2. It could help us feel a part of a community rather than a presence confined to an exam room.

I've also noticed that people often understand medical matters better when they are related as stories. When I prescribe steroids like prednisone, I like to tell clients the reason we often recommend a decreasing dose such as twice daily, then once daily, then every other day. I believe people are more likely to follow complicated instructions if they understand the logic—or story line—behind them.

"The reason is that Morrissey's body already manufactures steroids. When we supplement, his adrenal glands get the message that there's plenty available and his system then makes less. We want to give Morrissey a chance to ramp up production, which is why we don't like to stop this medication abruptly," I'll explain.

One owner looked at me in surprise. "I've been given steroids lots of times myself, and my doctors have never explained that to me. Thank you, now I understand."

As practitioners, when we hear our clients' stories, they become a part of our own stories of practice, of our daily lives, of respect and wonder at the ability of humans and animals to love each other and connect in a myriad of ways. Yet although I may be a part of a client and patient's story, and they a part of mine, their stories are not my own. Viewing my story as a narrative has helped me maintain healthier boundaries.

As we struggle to improve well-being in the veterinary profession and reduce burnout, compassion fatigue, and moral stress, narrative medicine could help us recognize where the narratives of our clients' end—and where our own stories begin.

I was so excited about narrative medicine that I wrote an article about it for a veterinary magazine. When I didn't see it in print, I contacted the publisher, who told me it was only available online. I was disappointed, as I'd worked hard on the article and wanted so badly to share the information with my colleagues. I didn't think many people would find it online.

Two years later, an unexpected email landed in my inbox. It was from an editor named Alice who worked for a well-known textbook publisher in London. The company was seeking someone to write a textbook on narrative medicine for veterinarians. Alice had read and enjoyed my online article. Would I be interested?

I was thrilled. I began reading more about narrative medicine in human medicine, and took many of my thoughts about practice I'd learned over the years from working with animals and clients and from talking things through with colleagues like Eileen. Something that especially concerned me was that, unlike human medicine, veterinary medicine doesn't have a tradition of reflection.

When I was in vet school, we were taught to get the job done and move on. We were not expected to think about ethical quandaries or the reasons we found a situation troubling. We were not taught self-compassion. Part of my goal in writing and teaching is to foster the ability to reflect in ways that were discouraged when I was in school. I want to show burgeoning veterinarians that they don't have to leave their humanity at the door if they want to be good doctors.

Recently there has been a realization among the medical and veterinary communities that we may be missing part of a bigger picture if we do not connect more with each other. Many physicians as well as laypeople are unaware of the similarities between human and animal physiology and disease. This is beginning to change, with the recent launch of an international effort called the One Health Initiative, which focuses on bringing together physicians and veterinarians along with environmentalists to consider the holistic health of the planet and its inhabitants.

Veterinarians are natural One Health practitioners. We are taught to extrapolate from human medicine, so we are aware of advances in human medical care and the ways animals can benefit from them. I had seen how the nomadic herders in Morocco lived in concert with their animals and their environment. Anything that affects animals, whether pets, livestock, or wild creatures, has the potential to affect people and the environment as well.

Unfortunately, despite the similarities in our vocations, there is currently no model for professional contact between physicians and veterinarians. Since those long-ago physiology classes and anatomy labs, I have had clients who are physicians and I have some physician relatives and friends. Otherwise, our worlds are separate.

Whenever I visit a new doctor as a patient, I always identify myself as a veterinarian, so the physician will know I understand medical terminology and concepts. After the physician enters the room and introduces themself, the conversation typically goes like this:

> **Me.** Just so you know, I'm a veterinarian. Okay, I've had this strange rash/eye floater/flu symptom since . . .
>
> **My doctor.** Oh, a veterinarian? Did you know veterinary school is harder to get into than medical school?
>
> **Me.** I have heard that, yes. There are fewer veterinary schools than medical schools. So, my symptoms started—
>
> **My doctor.** Hmm, I have a question for you. My eight-year-old Labradoodle just got diagnosed with Cushing's disease, and my wife and I are debating starting her on medication. What do you think?
>
> **Me.** Well, there are some pros and cons. Should I put the hospital johnny on open in the back or the front?

I have always found human doctors to be respectful; they seem to treat me as an unusual and interesting type of colleague. Certainly, no practicing physician has ever made farm-animal noises at me like the medical students did long ago. I do wonder sometimes how this parallel profession deals with the myriad of ethical and psychological issues both human and veterinary medical doctors face. Do they have more training than we do regarding difficult conversations? Do they internalize their feelings after giving a patient bad news? Are there things we can learn from each other? It seems unfortunate that we can no longer simply walk down a hallway, as we did during anatomy lab, and peer into the other's world.

I wish that physicians and veterinarians could more easily learn from each other about practice styles; for instance, we could share techniques to increase compliance among our patients and clients. We could compare strategies for self-care and wellness, setting boundaries, and handling the stress of conversations on mortality. Neither group is typically trained as therapists; while we can refer a person to a social worker, rarely is there one in the room with us when difficult topics are being discussed or bad news given.

With the emergence of Covid-19, One Health has become urgent. Veterinarians are critically important partners to scientists and physicians where zoonotic diseases, which can spread between humans and animals, are concerned. Some zoonotic diseases, like rabies, have been present for thousands of years and are still responsible for many deaths worldwide; others, like Covid-19 and Ebola, can develop from mutations. One Health will be important in the continuing surveillance to detect and control the development of further pandemics.

Many people are familiar with the adage about pets looking like their owners. Might animals also be susceptible to the same diseases as the humans in their household? I have frequently been surprised by the number of people who react to a pet's diagnosis with the disclosure that they, themselves, suffer from a similar condition. These are not zoonotic diseases; they are not contagious disorders at all. The complaints vary from cancer, thyroid disease, and diabetes to issues such as allergies, heart disease, and urinary tract infections.

One client confided to me that she hoped her cat did not have "the sugar," because she herself had diabetes. Blood tests proved the cat was indeed a diabetic. Another client called me to treat her cat's bladder infection. The client explained she had separated from her husband, was sleeping on a friend's couch, and both she and her cat had developed urinary tract infections as a response to the stress of the situation. A client whose dog had a swollen face from a tooth infection pulled out her phone to show me her own swollen face from the same problem two months earlier.

While the observations I've just described are purely anecdotal,

I am not the only veterinarian to notice that pets can appear to mirror their owners' health conditions. Scientists have begun to consider whether pets can serve as an early warning system for exposure to environmental hazards such as chemical pollutants in our homes and yards. One such possibility is that of cats and hyperthyroidism, as a study found that cats exposed to flame retardants commonly found on furniture suffered from a higher rate of thyroid disease. Another study found that people who owned a diabetic dog were more likely to develop diabetes than people who owned a nondiabetic dog.

As well as environmental factors, there could be other explanations why humans and animals who live together may develop similar health conditions. Perhaps humans and animals from the same household share similar microbiome organisms, which could make them susceptible to similar illnesses. Or could there be, as one client recently suggested to me, an energetic occurrence, some sort of transfer between species we do not yet understand? In Traditional Chinese Medicine, individuals are prone to certain conditions based on their constitution and other factors such as diet. Do we somehow choose pets who share our own tendencies and proclivities?

If the One Health model proves successful, the future will contain more connections between physicians, veterinarians, and environmentalists, and we can continue to explore the overlap between the professions as well as the responses of humans, animals, plants, and ecosystems to processes such as aging and disease, and identify the problems in parentheses as well as the more obvious issues.

One Health, it seems, could encompass more than the interconnection of human and animal health; examining the ways that animals approach illness and death may help us accept our own mortality.

23

I Fix Broken Hearts

The German shepherd's name was Duke, and it suited him well. Everything about him was large: his head, his body, his paws. When he entered the exam room, his long tongue hung down from his mouth as he panted (it was a hot day), and he took up so much space that it was hard to move around him. German shepherds are beautiful, intelligent, and loyal dogs, but they are not always the easiest patients to treat. Their intelligence can cause them to be wary and fearful if they feel threatened or haven't been properly socialized, and their size makes them difficult to handle if they are distressed. Some will even become "fear biters" and attack without warning if they feel cornered. Yet Duke was clearly friendly, relaxed, and enjoying the attention, so my assistant Michelle and I knew we didn't have to worry.

Michelle and I patted Duke's long black-and-tan fur, and he politely accepted a dog cookie from me. Without difficulty, we coaxed him onto the hydraulic exam table. Although some dogs balk at being raised up on the exam table, Duke didn't seem to mind at all. He took up the entire length. The table's scale showed he was well over a hundred pounds.

Duke's owner, Ed, was an older man with thinning gray hair. A younger man who may have been his son or grandson came with him, but Ed did the talking. Duke's bright eyes followed me as I checked his eyes and ears and felt around his neck for his lymph nodes. He allowed me to open his mouth and I commented on his worn teeth, recommending a different toy for chewing. German shepherds are known for being rock and tennis ball chewers and sometimes wear their teeth down to the gumline. I listened to Duke's heart as he leaned into Michelle, who was holding him still for me with one arm hugging his neck. Ed stood in front of Duke and spoke reassuringly to him. Michelle and I both commented on what a wonderful dog he was.

When I finished examining and vaccinating Duke, we lowered the table and fed him more treats. Then the young man fastened Duke's leash and took him out to the car. Michelle left the room to get the next patient's chart. It was just Ed and me in the exam room, which felt suddenly empty now that Duke wasn't there.

Ed sat down on one of the chairs to my right. "You know," he said, "before Duke, I had another shepherd, just as big—bigger even, than this one."

"Really?" I glanced at him with a smile before continuing to write medical notes in Duke's chart.

"Yes, and when he died, I was so upset. My wife, she told me I needed to get another one, and that's how I got Duke."

"That's great." I closed Duke's file. "Your wife knew how important he was to you."

Ed retrieved his wallet and opened it, searching. Suddenly, he froze. "I know you're busy, you have other patients to see . . ."

Warmth pulled at my heart. I knew this was where I needed to be; it didn't matter how busy I was. This was a part of Duke's story, and it was my job as his veterinarian to understand it. "I would love to see a picture."

Ed removed an old wallet-sized photo. It was worn at its edges and the color had faded. Yet Ed smiled as he looked at it. "This was Rex," he said proudly. The photo showed an enormous German shepherd standing in front of a ceiling-height Christmas tree. The dog took up half the picture.

"Oh, he's *beautiful*," I said. "He really was just as big."

"Do you know how I knew Duke was the right one? They both have the same spot on their side."

Duke was already in the car, so I peered at the photo again. "Where is the spot?"

"You can't see it in this picture; it's on his other side. But I couldn't believe, when I saw Duke, that he had the same spot."

Michelle came back into the room, and I called her over. She also examined the picture and exclaimed about the dog. It was a few moments before Ed was ready to tuck the photo back into his wallet and head out the door, happy to be reunited with Duke and yet still mourning the loss of Rex.

Ed had brought Duke in for a checkup, yet he had also wanted to talk about his previous dog. Taking the time to look at Rex's photo and recognize their relationship seemed nearly as important as Duke's wellness care. Rex remained significant enough to Ed that he carried the dog's picture in his wallet. And Ed still felt a connection to Rex through the spot on Duke's side.

I wondered how often Ed showed Rex's photo to people and considered the moment he had frozen, rethinking his decision. Had it been from embarrassment? Shame at being so attached to an animal that he carried a picture around, years after his dog's death?

For so many of us, for every pet that we love, there is another who lives on in our heart, who we can reach only through memories.

In addition to the love Mike and I shared with Rana, I have witnessed numerous love stories between human and animal, person and pet. Each one, unique and special. Each death, authentically grieved, the end of an era in someone's life.

If having a pet is one of life's great joys, then losing a pet is surely one of life's great sorrows. The two are inextricably linked, yin to yang, neither existing without the other. No joy without sorrow. No sorrow without joy.

Together, they merge, and form love.

Sometimes, this human-animal love is present in our lives but not central. We may have busy lives in which our pets are just a part. Perhaps we don't think of them as a fundamental presence, but they are there, as solid and reliable as a comfortable chair to sink into at the end of each day. Our pets bear witness to the intimate, everyday details of our daily existence, weaving and threading their own personalities into our lives and households. With them, we are home. When they are gone, we feel their absence deeply.

For others, or at certain times in one's life, the connection with their pet may be a central relationship, a primal bond. For a person living alone with few close human relationships, a pet may feel like their next of kin. However, the presence of other household members or close relationships in one's life does not immunize one against profound grief upon the death of a beloved pet. The connection can still be fundamental, the loss life-altering.

When I treat a pet with cancer, I sometimes explain to the owners that I was drawn to treat pets with cancer because of the large amount of information I gathered through researching Rana's care and treatment. I'll tell them I hope other animals can benefit from what I have learned. I may share how well she responded and how fully she lived, describing how she chased her tail, loved her walks, and ate with gusto even as the tumor continued to grow. I may even reveal a glimpse of my own struggle to accept her diagnosis. It was painful at first, but after some time, the anecdotes became well-traveled paths. I established some pieces of my experiences I felt comfortable sharing. I found that, as long as I stuck to my script, I was okay.

Yet, as I spend time with my clients and come to know the people and their animals better, things come up that are not in my safety zone. As I treat my animal patients with conventional Western medicine, Traditional Chinese Medicine, or a combination, I frequently sense that their owners—my clients—are in need as well. This is outside the scope of my training, but I am often faced with people who are in the midst of an emotional crisis. As I have learned to recognize patterns of disease and health in my patients, I have also learned to identify patterns of grief and hope in their human caretakers.

In our culture, medical professionals who treat humans generally hold themselves somewhat separate from the patients they treat. There are barriers not often crossed. Many physicians share little, if any, information about their own lives or thoughts about life. Such self-disclosure is usually discouraged as unprofessional. Veterinary medicine is different from human medicine, however. It is more earthy, less white-coat. I often find myself on the floor with my patients, meeting them at their level.

As I watch someone struggle with grief, acceptance, or decision-making, I find myself reaching back into my own suffering, searching for something—a memory, kind words, an insight—anything to help the brokenhearted person in front of me to at least realize they are not alone. Still, in doing so, I need to remain professional and maintain appropriate boundaries. I am not an ethicist, nor a psychologist; although I look to these fields often, my education in these disciplines has been on the fly. The last thing I wish to do is offend, so I speak in general terms as I mention a pet loss support hotline or describe how a similar situation was resolved. I don't say, "This will help you"; instead I offer, "This is something that helped me."

I didn't know there was a name for what I was doing. As it turns out, it is called self-disclosure, the sharing of personal feelings or stories with clients (or patients, in the human medical world). It is something I do reluctantly, a small sacrifice, the sharing of a painful story to help someone else. I say the words while trying not to relive the moment, disclosing the memory while holding it at arm's length.

I could not find anything written about self-disclosure in veterinary literature. It is not something I learned about in school. For physicians, there are a few journal articles exploring the topic, including a small study that revealed that although patients rated surgeons who self-disclosed more highly, they did not feel the same way about general practitioners. From the few articles I found, it appears physicians are not encouraged to self-disclose to their patients. Authors cautioned that self-disclosure should always be focused on the needs of the patient, never the doctor. *Better not to take a chance,* I read into the subtext. *Keep that boundary in place.*

I wonder whether pediatricians, those physicians whose work is arguably most closely related to veterinarians, self-disclose. Just as in veterinary medicine, there may exist many small opportunities. A veterinarian may say to a client, as a pediatrician may say to a parent, "Oh, I know what you mean. I have a hard time getting my own pet/child to take medication. Here are some things you can try," or even "This is what works for me."

Those little self-disclosures forge a connection, yet they tend to be easy and superficial. I'm not giving much away. The occasions when self-disclosure seems more important, and deeper, tend to involve the emotions around euthanasia and death, grief and loss, and decision-making after being issued a poor prognosis. When I see a person who is deeply upset, I want to give them permission to acknowledge their feelings.

I may tell someone that I made the decision to euthanize Trudy even though she was still eating. I revealed this to a client's adult son as he struggled with scheduling the appointment for his dog's euthanasia. It was part of a longer conversation, and I had been treating the dog for months. His mother, my client, later called to thank me. "What you said helped him," she said.

When I share something about myself, I try to let go of any personal objective for doing so. I do so because it *may* help, not because it *must* help. I put it out there, just in case. I don't seek any evidence of whether it brought comfort or not. Of course, it can be rewarding to know your words benefited someone. But I am fortunate; my clients often thank me profusely for my words and actions, so I am not in short supply of appreciation. Perhaps this allows me to be less invested in whether my words have supported an individual.

Perhaps the mere act of sharing a small, vulnerable piece of myself can benefit a client. After all, no two experiences are the same; even if our situations are similar, I cannot know what another is thinking or experiencing. What I can do is to let them know their struggles are common ones and that I struggled, too.

This extends to the decision to acquire another pet after one has died.

"That's it, I'm not getting another one," many people proclaim after the loss of a beloved cat or dog. "It's too painful. I can't go through this again." And yet, many of us do. We wait, some of us, a day, a month, a year or more, to open our hearts again. I may receive a phone call from a client or notice a familiar last name in the schedule at work. A new addition, bittersweet, but joyous, nonetheless. I smile, remembering, then look forward.

It can be a challenge to not feel guilty about acquiring another pet, to not regard it as an act of betrayal. I like to think of bringing a new pet into the home as a way to honor the memory of the previous one. I also like to consider that, metaphorically at least, the deceased animal had a hand in choosing the new one.

We sometimes see our old pet's behavior in the new one. "He's channeling Daiquiri," I used to think sometimes, when Marula gave a two-syllable meow. Of course, Marula was nothing like Daiquiri, either in looks or behavior. And Dai has been gone for many years now. And yet . . . naturally, there will occasionally be a similarity, a reminder of those who have gone before.

A few weeks after Rana's death, I was looking at puppies on Petfinder.com. Although I was still deeply grieving, I was finding it difficult to treat my canine patients and arrive home to a dog-free house. I had grown up without dogs and never wanted to be dogless again. I wasn't sure I was ready for another, but I had several factors to consider. I knew I wanted a puppy as our next dog, and winter was coming; it was November, and the weather grew colder as the days shortened. I didn't want to housebreak a puppy in snow, but I didn't want to wait until spring, either. So I began looking.

Mike was not in favor; he thought it was too soon. Everyone is different, I told him. I've seen clients wait months or years, and I've known people who've gone and adopted a new pet the very next day after losing one, knowing their previous friend could never be replaced but yearning for something to fill the void.

One day, I saw some adorable pictures of a litter of fuzzy black Lab mix puppies on a rescue website. I sent a brief email to the address on the website, asking whether the pups were local so I could meet them and mentioning that I was a veterinarian.

The response came quickly: no, the puppies were not local, they were in Indiana. The puppies had an interesting history, the email explained. They had been born in Louisiana before Hurricane Katrina went ashore in New Orleans. After Katrina, the puppies' owners were without power and were unable to care for them. The litter of pups was surrendered to a local rescue, which eventually sent them to a Lab rescue based in Indiana.

Of the litter, one special puppy, Anna (short for Louisiana—all the pups had names related to their birthplace), needed some extra attention. The veterinarian at the shelter had noticed a heart murmur, the email went on to say, and Anna had received an echocardiogram. She had been diagnosed with a condition called PDA, or patent ductus arteriosus. It was a serious heart problem, and little Anna would require surgery to live past puppyhood.

The ductus arteriosus is a small blood vessel outside the heart that is present while an animal or a person is in the womb and not breathing air. It normally closes within a few hours or days after birth. If it doesn't close naturally, it can be closed with surgery. A specialist performs the procedure, which typically resolves the problem, restoring the expectation of a normal life span for the affected animal. While Anna appeared healthy, she would need to have surgery soon to prevent the possibility of permanent heart problems and a shortened life span; many untreated animals live for less than one year.

The rescue was going to have the surgery performed on Anna, they informed me, but she wouldn't be adopted out until after she had recovered from the procedure—unless she happened to be adopted by a veterinarian. If Mike and I adopted Anna, we could nurse her through her recuperation from heart surgery.

Mike and I discussed the matter for a few days as I corresponded with the rescue group, and he and I went back and forth about a decision. "Can't we get a normal, *healthy* pet?" he asked reasonably. Yes, the picture was adorable, he acknowledged. But after everything we had gone through with Rana, Mike didn't want to risk getting attached to an animal with medical problems. "Haven't we had enough medical issues to deal with?" he asked.

"Vets don't have 'normal' pets," I responded. I knew Mike had a point. Yet this was a medical problem with a high likelihood of a complete cure.

There was no question whether I was still moping around after Rana's death. I knew life would never be the same without her. The puppy would be a good diversion, I figured, a reason (in addition to Marula) to fill the water bowl every day. Someone to take for walks. I wanted—*needed*—some canine energy in the house. But would it be fair to this new puppy, I asked myself, to bring her into our home while I was still so sad? When would I *not* be sad? I sat down at the computer and looked at the puppy's picture again, staring at the screen for a few moments, trying to read the future in her photo. Finally, I turned off the computer. It was time to go to work at the clinic; time to care for other people's dogs and cats.

I went outside and got into my car. As I turned the key in the ignition, music came on, the radio station playing a song and artist I knew well. As the meaning of the words filtered into my mind, my eyes widened and filled with tears. I froze, listening.

"*I fix broken hearts, I know that I truly can,*" sang James Taylor.

It was the song "Handy Man." That's it, I thought: Mike and I have broken hearts, and this puppy has a broken heart. She needs us, and our hearts can heal together. I sat in the car and cried.

I knew what Mike would say when I told him about the song; I could picture his eye roll. But I had my sign. Things weren't perfect—I would still rather have Rana than any other dog in the world. But I would open my heart and home to another dog. I would take care of a puppy who needed surgery, and maybe she would take care of me and Mike, too.

———

We named our little puppy Velvet, and she survived her heart surgery and grew to be a sweet and happy girl. Although she looked dainty, with her slim muzzle and delicate paws, she was the alpha when she played with other dogs, her favorite activity. Even Mike agreed that she needed a friend, so we adopted an adult Lab mix, Remy, from the same rescue; his name was short for Velvet's Remedy, and the two became inseparable. Remy was sturdy with an athletic build, yet he loathed going outside in bad weather or even onto wet grass. Velvet was unfazed by rain, snow, and wind—after all, we figured, she had been born during a hurricane.

Marula spent many years getting into trouble. He had a special relationship with my son, beginning during my pregnancy, when he would snuggle up to my belly and purr. He also liked to sit next to me while I wrote, but he too is now gone. New animals have come to live with and love us; they can never replace the ones that have gone before, but we love them, too.

Rana, I know, would be gone now, even if she had not been diagnosed with her aggressive cancer, even if she had lived to be a very old dog. Although she lived to be only five years old, she lived six times longer than the oncologist had predicted. She spent over one-quarter of her life with cancer. I still think of the Rana-Colored Thread, and I think of Rana often. She remains a part of my life, as strange as that may sound. Sometimes at night, if I can't sleep, I'm upset about something, or I don't feel good, I think of her. I picture, in my mind's eye, Rana jumping onto the bed and curling up by my feet, nose to crooked tail. I can't pat her soft ears anymore, nor laugh at her cute antics, but I am reminded that her spirit is in my heart as surely as it ever was, and I am calmed. I can almost feel the weight of her body, her love surrounding and sheltering me, and I know she is with me still.

The human-animal bond varies not only from person to person but from creature to creature, and I have had a unique bond with each animal that has shared my home. Each pet has had their own narrative both as an individual and as a part of my own story. I've also been a small part of the stories of my patients and clients: Dick and Claire and Arnell the pig; Miles the feral cat who held out his paw so I could trim his nail; Ed and his German shepherd Rex, a dog I knew only through viewing his photo. My grandfather, too, has accompanied me as I follow his path of home visits and discover my patients' narratives. The stories connect us all.

In my work, I have been privileged to have met many interesting people and many wonderful cats and dogs. The greatest blessings I've received, though, are the glimpses of the wonderful threads that connect them—and I have seen threads of all shapes, sizes, and colors. If you observe carefully, you may realize the universe is alive with threads; they glisten in the sun, and they are always there, remaining intact through the long nights, through the storms and the winters and the dry heat of summer. And although they may fade, they do not disappear.

24

Learning from Animals

My own cancer, diagnosed years after Rana's death, was found on a routine mammogram and came as a complete surprise.

Directly after my diagnosis, flowers, cards, and candy arrived at the house daily. My phone rang continuously, as friends and family members called to hear my voice and to offer support. At one point, I answered the phone to hear Lisa saying, annoyed, "You know, you're much harder to get hold of now that you have cancer!" Her comment had me laughing for days. Lisa went to some of my appointments with me, taking notes as she had done when we met with Rana's oncologist.

Unlike Rana's, my tumor was able to be surgically removed shortly after diagnosis. As I subsequently received first chemotherapy and then radiation treatments, I discovered I felt the same way about my own tumor cells as I had about Rana's. I did not feel I was waging a battle. I felt I was doing everything possible to convince any rogue cells in my body to take one for the team.

The cancer and I went to mediation.

Yes, it was tough, and I had to be strong. But perhaps due to my training and experience as a holistic doctor, I personally could not relate to the classic warrior metaphor. Maybe I was being a warrior, but if so, I was doing it in another way. I concluded that, as with many things in life, there is no one right way to think about cancer.

Surprisingly, my sense of humor, which had been in short supply during Rana's care, came to the fore. It was easier to find something funny when it was myself who was affected, I discovered, rather than a loved one. Our son, Nate, was born three years after Rana died, and he was then three years old. Having a preschooler around helped me keep my sense of perspective.

One of the first people who came to mind after my diagnosis was my friend Janet's son, Stephen. Diagnosed with leukemia two years earlier at age ten, he had already been through two years of chemo, with another one and a half to go. *If Stephen can have chemo for three years*, I resolved, *I can do it for three months.*

The other person I knew who'd had chemo was a veterinary technician from the clinic, Caelyn. Then in her midtwenties, she had survived ovarian cancer diagnosed when she was a teenager. Occasionally when Caelyn was in the exam room helping me with a patient, a client would mention that they or a loved one was undergoing chemotherapy. Sometimes they would whisper the word *chemo*, especially older clients. "Oh, I've had chemo," Caelyn would comment as she held their pet, making no attempt to lower her voice as she said the word. She discussed chemo as if it were any other unpleasant medical procedure, and cancer with gravity yet also with a casual nonchalance. She was honest and open about her experiences, and I watched many clients visibly relax as she conversed with them.

Especially since I practice holistic medicine, I meet many people who recoil from the word *chemo*, equating it with poison, and I've resolved to not consider it so negatively. Just the word *chemo* made the side effects seem worse, I mused on a good day; if I didn't think of the C word, my side effects felt like a combination of a mild flu on top of early pregnancy symptoms, with a few other unpleasantries (like mouth sores) thrown in for good measure.

I considered the many animals I have seen receive chemo while exhibiting minimal side effects. Although I've never worked at an animal hospital that uses chemotherapeutic agents, I have treated many patients while they were receiving chemotherapy through oncologists at another hospital. I knew that chemo constitutes many different types of drugs and combinations of drugs; the side effects from one chemo regimen may be different from those of another, not to mention the differences between individuals. I have seen some animals not feel well on chemo protocols, causing their owners to discontinue their treatment. Yet I have seen many more animals do well, with few side effects. I do believe dogs and cats benefit from not having the mental stress that people tend to have when we hear the dreaded words *cancer* and *chemo*. Animals are not worried about short- or long-term side effects, when they can return to work, or how on earth they are going to pay for all this.

Along with my sense of humor, and support from friends and family near and far, something else helped me through cancer treatment: a class called Mindfulness-Based Stress Reduction, or MBSR, a concept initiated by Jon Kabat-Zinn at the University of Massachusetts Medical School, located just a few miles from my home. It was the hospital that Rana had run to and where she was scooped up and saved by Rocky the valet. It was also the hospital where I was getting my cancer treatment. But my recommendation to MBSR came from across the world—it was my aunt Sue in Brisbane, Australia, who suggested it to me via email. She had taken the course, and it had helped her deal with some medical issues she was having.

After my oncologist said I would have to stop working for several months due to an increased risk of infection in my profession, I decided to do something for myself during that time. It might have been a pottery class, but, due to my aunt's gentle but repeated urgings, I investigated the MBSR class. It turned out there was a new session starting just as I was scheduled to begin chemo. The class met for three hours once a week for several weeks. The structure sounded good to me at a time when the rest of my life felt chaotic, and I signed up.

The course alternated between discussion, yoga, meditation, and explanations of this thing called mindfulness—otherwise known as being in the moment. Why is it, our class explored, that so often our minds are misaligned with our bodies, our thoughts either repeating past events or imagining future ones, rather than remaining in the present? What does this mean about how we live our lives? I had tried to embrace the Serenity Prayer during Rana's treatment, but although I agreed with the principle of it, I had found myself unable to follow it. The MBSR class, building on my previous yoga training, gave me the tools I needed to incorporate the sentiments of the Serenity Prayer into my daily life so that I could let go of some of the things I couldn't control.

One of the hardest parts of chemo was the hair loss, as it felt in a primal way as though my body was unraveling. Like many women, I'd had a love-hate relationship with my hair. It may not have been the hair I would have chosen, but I'd accepted it. I'd taken care of it every day, like a pet; since childhood I had brushed it, washed it, played with it. Knowing it would soon be gone, I wrapped my hair around my hand as I lay in bed at night, holding on to it while I still could.

When my hair began to fall out, friends offered to come over and shave it off. I'd read that it was better to shave one's head rather than experience a slow, continuous loss, so I agreed. We decided to try to make it a happy occasion, particularly for Nate's sake.

The day of the shave, I brought Nate to our favorite bakery, Wholly Cannoli, to choose a selection of mini pastries, something that always made me happy. As we waited in line at the busy counter, I glanced down to see Nate spread-eagled on the display case in front of us, face against the glass, tongue out and glued to the window to get as close as possible to the goodies below. Nate knew his mom was sick; years later, he still gets upset if I contract the slightest cold. But at that moment, he was one with the cannoli, which made me laugh and laugh.

The hair loss also made my diagnosis more public. I preferred to wear headscarves, after concluding that the wig I'd ordered looked better than my real hair (thus causing me to anticipate fielding comments regarding a new hairstyle) and was scratchy and uncomfortable besides.

The support from friends and family was invaluable, but ultimately it was my body and me, alone, who had to face the physical and mental challenges. On the bad days, this led to a feeling of isolation, as though I were alone on an island. Fortunately, I could communicate with other people who were alone on other islands. As hard as it was to leave the house with a scarf covering my bald head, it was wonderful to have a stranger come up to me and wish me luck, confiding that they had been there, too.

Remy, Velvet, and Marula also seemed to understand, keeping me company as I rested from the effects of treatment. One rainy day, I stood at the door to our fenced dog yard. Velvet was already outside, but Remy refused to go. "Remy," I told him, "if I can have chemo, you can pee in the rain." He went.

Feeling restless and uneasy the day before one of my chemo treatments, I left Mike and Nate at home and drove to a place that felt like a sanctuary: a bookstore, where I chose some reading material for the days ahead. Next door was a coffee shop; it was a hot day, and I went in to order a lemonade before sitting at one of the outdoor tables. As I waited, I noticed some chocolate chip cookies behind the counter, and I asked the young man who was helping me to add one to my order. At the register, I was handed the drink and the cookie but charged only for the drink. When I tried to tell him I'd been undercharged, he waved me away.

That cookie, flavored with the kindness of a stranger, fortified me for the days ahead.

On another day, Mike commented, "You look tired."

"Nuh-uh," I responded confidently. "Today three people told me I look good!"

Mike just looked at me.

"*Ohhh,*" I said slowly, eyes widening as the realization hit me. "You mean . . . they think I look good *for someone who is having chemo.*" I thought for a minute, frowning in concentration. It was hard not to get a swelled head, walking around and having everyone tell you how good you looked all the time. The shock came when you looked in the mirror.

I have fallen into the same trap myself, even after undergoing chemo. When I see someone after a cancer diagnosis or who is going through chemo, my first urge is to tell them how good they look. Although, maybe that isn't a bad thing. If people think you are awesome just for leaving the house or getting out of bed during a difficult time, maybe that's okay.

One evening during my treatment, I put my son to bed. I sang to him and rubbed his back. I was physically in the room with him, but my mind was far away. *What if the cancer comes back and spreads?* I was thinking.

Suddenly, with a jolt, I realized I was not being mindful. My body was here, having a pleasant moment with my son, in his cozy room filled with stuffed animals, books, and little-boy things. It should have been a nice time of day, bonding with my sleepy child, knowing some "me" time would come afterward, and I could unwind and spend time with my husband. Yet I was not calm and relaxed. Instead, my mind was in a very unpleasant place.

I pushed the thought further. I wondered, what if the cancer *did* come back, and I had denied myself the enjoyment of this nice moment with my son? How would that help? The worrying drained me, I realized, and deprived me of happiness and relaxation. Perhaps, I concluded, I would be better off appreciating these special moments. Maybe they would even have a fortifying effect, if indeed I were to face the challenge of a recurrence. I thought of Daiquiri. I thought of Trudy. I thought of Rana.

I used to believe, deep down, that there was preventive power in the simple act of worrying. Whenever my mind spun elaborate tales of Things That Could Go Wrong, I dutifully followed along, carrying the belief that something about my thoughts was helpful and productive; that if I only worked and worried hard enough, I could insulate myself against the possibility of disaster.

Now I have changed my philosophy. I still think ahead and worry, but I try to do so only enough to make any preparations I may need. Worrying does not aid in the mental preparation for adversity. I know that when disasters do come, they do not look like I thought they would, as was the case with four-year-old Rana, and I will need the courage and strength to think on my feet. The best way to prepare for those moments in the future is to be present in the way that animals are present.

I am grateful for all I have learned from animals—from watching wild animals on safari, from seeing how the lives of nomadic herders in Morocco were intertwined with those of their sheep, from connecting with people over their love for their pets, and from sharing my life with my own animal companions. Animals connect us to the environment, as Trudy did when I walked her in the woods; to our families, as Rana's care deepened my connections with Mike and Lisa; and to our own reactions to illness and death, as Rana taught me about living with cancer and Daiquiri about accepting mortality. After Rana's and my cancers, I know that growing older, while not always easy, is a blessing, and I am happy even for the challenges it brings.

That's why we love creatures who will not outlive us. That's why we put our hearts on the line for them, why we avoid travel to be with them, why we spend our savings to keep them healthy, why we deal with all the messes and all the hassle. Because doing so teaches us about being human.

Loving animals teaches us about being alive.

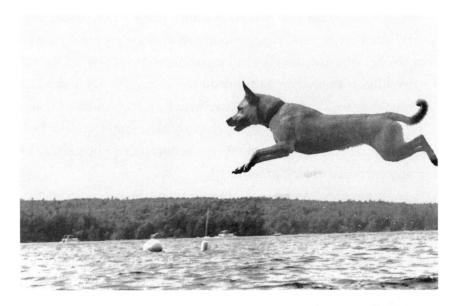

Acknowledgments

Thank you to all the wonderful people at Anchor Books, especially my amazing editor, Anna Kaufman, who warmly welcomed *The Other Family Doctor* into the perfect forever home. Thank you to Megan Wilson, Kayla Overbey, copy editor Shasta Clinch, proofreaders Hayley Jozwiak and Robin Witkin, text designer Nicholas Alguire, publicist Julie Ertl, and marketer Annie Locke. I've long been a fan of illustrator Iain MacIntosh, who creates covers for Alexander McCall Smith, and I'm beyond thrilled that he designed the gorgeous cover!

I'm very grateful to my literary agent, Jenny Herrera, who understood the book from the very beginning. Thank you to all who read early drafts and provided feedback, including Mike Dziura, David Fine, Angela Fine, Celia Fine, Eileen Mulcahy, Tom Dyer, Hazel Rochman, Maddy Wilks, Cheryl Dziura Duke, Sky E. Burr-Drysdale, and Hugh McElaney. Thank you to the Seven Bridge Writers' Collaborative and critique group members Paula Castner,

Bob Ainsworth, Andrew Linnell, Jill Andrews, Maureen Power, and Savi Fitch. Thank you to rock star editor Allison K. Williams and her life-changing writing retreats! Thank you to Dinty W. Moore and all the attendees of Rebirth Your Book Certaldo 2019 and 2021, especially writer and photographer Constance Owens. Thank you to the Binders.

Thank you to all the amazing veterinarians I've been fortunate to know and work with, including mentors Carolyn Prouty, Robin Chapman, Bart Murphy, Carlos E. Silvera, Steve Marsden, and Eileen Mulcahy. Eileen, thank you for your friendship, for being my animals' doctor, and for so many discussions about life, death, and everything in between! Thank you to all my colleagues and coworkers at Central Animal Hospital in Leominster, Massachusetts. I love veterinary medicine, even though it's not all puppy breath and roses. I hope more veterinarians and staff tell their stories, and I believe narrative medicine can help us do that. Thank you to the growing veterinary narrative medicine community, including Monica Mansfield, Jamie Falzone, Alice Oven, Sonja Olson, Michele Gaspar, and especially Annie Wayne, who had the brilliant idea of creating a veterinary NM journal, *Reflections*. Thank you to my alma mater, Tufts, and to John Bourgeois for your research assistance. Thank you to my own doctor, Deb Ford, who has my oupa's touch.

I'm so grateful to my dear friends—I can't imagine life without you! Lisa Weinberg, Janet Ruggieri, Karen Richter-Hall, Robin Blumenthal, Elizabeth Murphy, Maddy Wilks, Lisa Schwartz, Stephanie Ruggiere, and Dina Tedeschi (who also happens to be a website whiz). Thank you to Bob and Melanie Paradise for the Big Shave and for helping with Arnell! And big thanks to my extended family, including cousins Simon Rochman, Janine Stephen, Joanne Freedman, and my incredible aunts Hilary, Sue, Joy, and Hazel, who has sent me books all my life. Thank you to Mike's wonderful family for accepting me as their own. And in loving memory of my grandparents, my uncle Hymie, and my mother-in-law, Laurette.

Thank you to my mother for raising a reader and to my favorite and only brother for being a great sibling (even though he wasn't a puppy) and for providing emergency tech support. Dad and Angela, a million thanks for your endless support and encouragement; it has meant the world to me. And, of course, Mike and Nate, thank you for all your help, including all the times you had to listen to writing and publishing talk and the many times you brought me chocolate! Toffee, Sesame, and Lilac, you've been wonderful emotional support animals to us all.

I would like to acknowledge that this book was written on the traditional homeland of the Nipmuc people.

Finally, thank you to all the clients and patients I've met over the years, those in the book and the many who aren't. It's a privilege to be part of your stories. Special thanks to those who send thank-you and holiday cards and who bring food and gifts into the clinic; it sustains us more than you know.

To everyone who has bonded deeply with an animal, this book is for you.

Rituals for Grieving
the Loss of a Pet

I believe it is important that we grieve fully for our animal friends after they die. When we have shared a profound bond, a deep relationship with another creature, it *matters*, whether or not they were human. There are many different traditions and rituals that people have developed to mourn for humans, and some of these can be appropriated for pets.

Many people set up a temporary informal shrine in their homes, with pictures, a candle, a toy, a collar, and perhaps some fur or other mementos. When children are involved, it can be helpful to have a family circle and share stories about the pet.❝ Some people light a candle or have a moment of silence.

If you choose to bury the body or ashes, you may wish to have a small funeral service. Choose a time of day when you don't have to rush off to work or school. You can have a moment of silence or have anyone who wants to say a few words.

❝ See "How to Write a Pet Obituary" on page 281 for ideas of what to talk about.

A Celebration of Life is sometimes done for people and can easily be adapted for our animal friends. After our dog Remy died, we brought an ice-cream sundae party to the clinic where I worked, as he had been hospitalized there for several days before he died and my coworkers took excellent care of him. My son shared a slideshow he had made about Remy's life.

Try not to expect anything from others in your family; different people grieve in different ways, and at different times. I do believe, however, that it is important to acknowledge our grief, and to confide in people who understand.

How to Write a Pet Obituary

There is no right or wrong way to write an obituary for your pet. The goal is to put something down on paper—or computer—to memorialize your beloved animal, and your relationship. No memory is too small or insignificant; it is the tiny intimate details many people miss most. You can do this individually or together with other family members or friends. You can do it a little at a time or all at once. You can make your obituary as high tech (all computerized) or as low tech (handwritten) as you choose, but I do recommend that you print out a copy if you write something on the computer, so you have something tangible and real, rather than solely virtual.

There is also no right or wrong time to write about your pet. Even if they died many years ago, it may still be helpful to write an obituary for them.

Here are some ideas of what to write about to get you started:

- Write out a list of your pet's nicknames (possibly including how they came to be).

+ How did you obtain your pet? Describe the first time you saw them.

+ Who do they leave behind? Include family, any other animals, and friends.

+ Did you know your pet as a puppy, a kitten, or a young animal? What was your pet like as a youngster, or when they first came to live with you?

+ What were your pet's favorite games, toys, and activities?

+ What was your pet's favorite food?

+ What places did your pet travel to? What was their favorite place to visit?

+ Where was your pet's favorite place to sleep?

+ What was your pet's favorite time of year?

+ What was your favorite part of your daily routine with your pet?

+ Describe your pet's personality, including good and bad qualities (i.e., sneaking food off the counters). What mischief did your pet get into?

+ What were your favorite personality traits and quirks?

Once you have created something, here are some ideas for what to do with your pet obituary.

You can email your writing to friends and family or post it online on social media to let people know about your loss. You may then wish to invite people to share their own memories of your pet. You can also send a copy to your veterinarian, groomer, pet store owner, doggie day care provider, dog walker, or anyone else who has been a part of your pet's life.

You can print out or create a copy of your pet's obituary and put it somewhere in your home along with a picture of your pet, a candle, a favorite toy, and any other mementos to create a small shrine. If you choose, you can purchase special, decorative printer paper to print your words onto. You can frame a copy, or place one in a drawer or with your pet's ashes if you have chosen to keep them. You can keep a copy with you, in your pocket or in your wallet or purse.

If you have children, you can give them each their own copy, and they can decide where they would like to keep it. They may choose to personalize their copy with drawings or additional words.

If you choose to make a donation in your pet's memory, you may choose to include a copy of your pet's obituary.

RANA'S OBITUARY

Rana died peacefully at home today surrounded by family. Although she was only five and a half years old, she lived a very full life and gave and received a long lifetime's worth of love.

I first saw Rana on May 1, 2000, when she was brought into the animal hospital by the shelter after being hit by a car (two, actually) the day before. The instant I touched her, I felt like the Grinch at the end of the story when his heart grows three sizes that day.

We seemed instantly connected and I knew I had to bring her home with me.

Rana had what we call in Traditional Chinese Medicine a "Fire" personality. She was joyous every single day. She loved life and experienced every moment fully. She was like a bright light in our lives. She was mischievous, too, always trying to sneak some food or get into trouble. She made us laugh every day. She was also incredibly loving. Mike called her the "empathy dog" because she was always right there if one of us was upset. She'd sit in front of you, then rest her paws on you and balance while she gazed at you with round eyes full of concern. Or she'd find your hand and literally place her head under it, as if to say, *Pat me, you'll feel better.* Her favorite place to be was curled up at our feet.

Rana seemed to be one of those dogs that has nine lives like a cat. She escaped with only two broken toes after being hit by the two cars. When she was still a puppy, she managed to wiggle her way out of the fenced-in backyard (that Trudy had never escaped from) and disappeared. I was beside myself. We found out that she ran about three miles along a busy road, then crossed a divided highway to end up at the hospital, where a kindly valet rescued her. He put her in his truck and called the dog officer. When I came to get her, she didn't have a scratch on her. (I sent all the valets pizza with a card saying that they saved my puppy from being "road pizza.")

For me, one of the best parts of Rana's life was watching Mike fall in love with her. He went from being dog phobic to being just as attached to her as I was. She adored him and followed him wherever he went. Of course, we'll never forget her standing beside us at our wedding as the Dog of Honor (and interspecies representative). She loved all the socializing and picture-posing involved.

Rana's cancer diagnosis made us all even more attached. I was utterly devastated . . . but determined to do whatever I could to keep her healthy. We began home cooking for her, and I spent hours and hours researching holistic cancer treatment. Mike took on the task of grinding her vegetables and helped me each week to assemble her medications into daily portions (she took over a dozen herbs and supplements at each meal). We could never have done this without all the advice and support of some of the world's most talented veterinarians, who were all extremely generous with their time and knowledge, as well as the support of our friends and family.

Rana blossomed with all the special care. Her tumor continued to grow, but the rest of her was in great shape. We took her everywhere—on vacation in Maine, camping weekends, the beaches on Cape Cod, the Berkshires, family cookouts, long walks, swimming, even dog agility class—and she had a great time. The oncologists at Tufts had given her a prognosis of three months (eight if we did radiation, which we elected not to do for quality-of-life issues because the cancer was on her face), and she lived for eighteen. Just over the last few weeks, the now-enormous tumor was starting to bother her. Despite painkillers, she began to rub continually at her face, and despite a miraculous Chinese herbal medicine to stop bleeding (which had helped for months), she was bleeding every day.

Our home and hearts are rich with memories. We can still see her chasing her crooked little tail (and the way she would look at it first, like it was taunting her), swimming after ducks in the lake, and snoozing on the sofa with her head on her favorite Scooby-Doo pillow. It's just hard to know, though, that we'll never pat that soft fur again or see the light and concern in her eyes. I'm going to miss the weight of her lying on my feet . . . but I know she's there.

Resources

Further Reading and Information

- General veterinary information: veterinarypartner.com

- My article in *The Bark* magazine about handling a difficult diagnosis: "Ten Tips for Navigating Tough Decisions about Your Dog," October 2018, thebark.com/content/10-tips -navigating-tough-decisions-about-your-dog

- My article in *The Bark* magazine about how we grieved for Remy: "A Vet Gives Wise Counsel About Grieving (Or, How I Mourned My Own Dog)," June 2018, thebark.com /content/vet-gives-wise-counsel-about-grieving

- *Zoobiquity: The Astonishing Connection Between Human and Animal Health* by Barbara Natterson-Horowitz and Kathryn Bowers

One Health Initiative

+ onehealthinitiative.com

+ American Veterinary Medical Association's One Health page: avma.org/kb/resources/reference/pages/one-health .aspx

Pet Loss

Books for Adults

+ *Good Grief: On Loving Pets, Here and Hereafter* by E. B. Bartels is an enjoyable and comforting read about the different ways people (including the author) have memorialized their pets.

+ *P.S. I Love You More Than Tuna* by Sarah Chauncey is a gift book for adults who have lost a cat; it's also appropriate for children grieving a cat they helped to care for.

+ *The Pet Loss Companion* by Ken Dolan-Del Vecchio and Nancy Saxton-Lopez was written by family therapists who've led pet loss groups.

+ *Goodbye, Friend: Healing Wisdom for Anyone Who Has Ever Lost a Pet* by Gary Kowalski; Kowalski is a Unitarian Universalist minister.

+ *Coping with Sorrow on the Loss of Your Pet* by Moira Anderson Allen, MEd

+ *When Your Pet Dies: A Guide to Mourning, Remembering and Healing* by Alan D. Wolfelt, PhD

+ *The Loss of a Pet: A Guide to Coping with the Grieving Process When a Pet Dies* by Wallace Sife, PhD

Books for Children

+ *The End of Something Wonderful: A Practical Guide to a Backyard Funeral* by Stephanie V. W. Lucianovic is a direct and funny book about saying goodbye to different kinds of animals.

+ *The Goodbye Book* by Todd Parr is about a fish who has lost his fish companion and the range of emotions he experiences.

+ *Sally Goes to Heaven* by Stephen Huneck is one in a series of beautifully illustrated books about a black Labrador named Sally.

+ *The Invisible Leash* by Patrice Karst is about an invisible leash that feels like love.

+ *Cat Heaven* (there's also a *Dog Heaven*) by Cynthia Rylant; Rylant is the author of the Henry and Mudge children's book series.

+ *The Tenth Good Thing About Barney* by Judith Viorst

+ *When a Pet Dies* by Fred Rogers

Support Websites

In addition to the following websites, many veterinary school websites have resource pages.

+ In Memory of Pets, a memorial and tribute site: in-memory
  -of-pets.com

+ Monday Pet Loss Candle Ceremony: petloss.com

+ Rainbows Bridge, a virtual memorial home and grief
  support community: rainbowsbridge.com

+ The Pet Loss Support Page: pet-loss.net

+ Association for Pet Loss and Bereavement: aplb.org

Hotlines

Pet loss hotlines are offered by many veterinary schools as well as other organizations. Most are staffed part-time and will state their hours when you call. You can leave a message and your call will be returned when they are next staffed.

+ ASPCA (American Society for the Prevention of Cruelty
  to Animals): 877- GRIEF-10 (877-474-3310)

+ Chicago Veterinary Medical Association: 630-325-1600

+ Cornell University School of Veterinary Medicine:
  607-218-7457

+ Cummings School of Veterinary Medicine at Tufts
  University: 508-839-7966

Finding a New Pet

Pet Adoption

+ *The Doggie in the Window* by Rory Kress takes a deep dive into the world of puppy mills.

+ The Humane Society of the United States details how to avoid purchasing a dog from a puppy mill and provides information on how we can work to end puppy mills: humanesociety.org/all-our-fights/stopping-puppy-mills

+ Petfinder is a user-friendly website that allows searches by region as well as by breed, age, size, and many other characteristics: petfinder.com

+ The Shelter Pet Project, sponsored by the Humane Society of the United States, connects people with adoptable pets and shelters in their areas: theshelterpetproject.org

How to Find a Good Breeder

If you must purchase a puppy from a breeder, please read the excellent web article from the Humane Society of the United States, "How to Find a Responsible Dog Breeder": humanesociety.org /issues/puppy_mills/tips/finding_responsible_dog_breeder .html.

In short:

+ A reputable breeder cares more about the puppies they place than about their bank balance (or yours).

+ They will try to match the puppy's personality to your home environment to assure a good match, rather than allowing a buyer to choose according to a preferred color or gender.

+ The puppies will have been born on-site, and you will meet at least one of the parents, who will be friendly and healthy. The breeder will happily welcome you to their home and will not pressure you to instead meet them in a parking lot or to have the puppy shipped to you directly.

+ Most importantly, a good breeder will want you to surrender the dog back to them if you cannot care for it at some point in the animal's life, ensuring that the puppies they place will never end up unclaimed in a shelter.

Care for Pets

Clicker Training
Karen Pryor's website is clickertraining.com and contains a wealth of information.

Home Cooking for Pets
Home cooking should *always* be done under veterinary supervision, while following a recipe, so check with your veterinarian first. Otherwise the diet may not be safe for long-term use.

+ BalanceIT® provides recipes that are complete if you purchase their supplements (if you prefer, you can use your own supplements and purchase a recipe): balanceit.com

+ JustFoodForDogs also provides supplements and recipes: justfoodfordogs.com

Veterinary Acupuncture
Both the AAVA (American Academy of Veterinary Acupuncture) and the IVAS (International Veterinary Acupuncture Society) provide searchable databases of veterinary acupuncturists by region.

+ American Academy of Veterinary Acupuncture: aava.org

+ International Veterinary Acupuncture Society: ivas.org

+ *Four Paws, Five Directions: A Guide to Chinese Medicine for Cats and Dogs* by Cheryl Schwartz, DVM

Care for Humans

MBSR (Mindfulness-Based Stress Reduction)

+ UMass Memorial Health Center for Mindfulness: ummhealth.org/center-mindfulness

Veterinary Social Work

+ University of Tennessee, Knoxville's Veterinary Social Work: vetsocialwork.utk.edu

Suicide Prevention and Mental Health Resources
Many thanks to Dr. Bree Montana of Vets4Vets® for compiling the following resources and granting permission to share it.

+ Vets4Vets® is a confidential support service provided by the VIN Foundation. It's available at no cost to veterinarians and veterinary students anywhere in the world. Vet-

erinarians can call (530) 794-8094 or email Vets4Vets@
VINFoundation.org. Support staff can email Support4
Support@VINFoundation.org.

+ The 988 Suicide & Crisis Lifeline provides a free, anonymous
  connection, available 24/7, for those feeling suicidal, as well
  as for anyone concerned that someone they know may be
  suicidal. Call or text 988, or visit 988lifeline.org.

+ Crisis Text Line provides free, fast, anonymous, 24/7
  crisis support. Simply text "HOME" to 741741. Visit
  crisistextline.org for more.

+ Find your local chapter of the American Foundation for
  Suicide Prevention: afsp.org

+ IMAlive offers a free, anonymous, online chat option for
  those in need, as well as resources that may help diffuse
  anxiety and dissipate pressure and loneliness: imalive.org

+ Learn the warning signs of suicide and what you can do to
  help yourself and others: stopasuicide.org

+ The Center for Disease Control's "Suicide Prevention
  Resource for Action" is a printable prevention resource for
  communities: cdc.gov/suicide/pdf/preventionresource.pdf

+ The National Wellness Institute provides a variety of
  assessments: nationalwellness.org/testwell/twfree.htm

+ The HeartMath Institute's Personal Well-Being Survey™
  measures four key elements of well-being (stress
  management, adaptability, resilience, and emotional vitality):
  heartmath.org/resources/personal-well-being-survey

About the Author

Dr. Karen Fine is a holistic veterinarian who is fascinated by the relationships between animals and their people. She is an associate veterinarian at Central Animal Hospital in Leominster, Massachusetts. For twenty-five years she owned and operated her own house call practice in central Massachusetts. Dr. Fine is certified in veterinary acupuncture through the International Veterinary Acupuncture Society. A leading expert in the emerging field of veterinary narrative medicine, she has also authored a textbook called *Narrative Medicine in Veterinary Practice*.

karenfinedvm.com